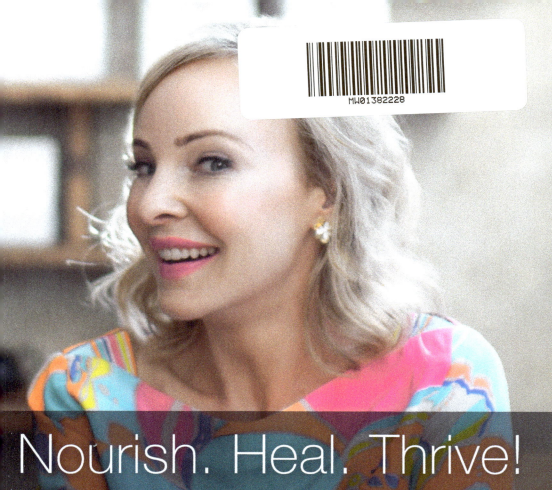

# Nourish. Heal. Thrive!
your path to vibrant health + radiant beauty

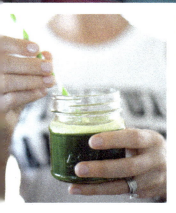
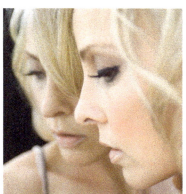
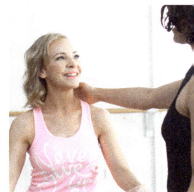

## Heather Hudak

Nourish. Heal. Thrive!
*Your* Path to Vibrant Health + Radiant Beauty
All Rights Reserved.
Copyright © 2020 Heather Hudak
v3.0

The opinions expressed in this manuscript are solely the opinions of the author and do not represent the opinions or thoughts of the publisher. The author has represented and warranted full ownership and/or legal right to publish all the materials in this book.

This book may not be reproduced, transmitted, or stored in whole or in part by any means, including graphic, electronic, or mechanical without the express written consent of the publisher except in the case of brief quotations embodied in critical articles and reviews.

Outskirts Press, Inc.
http://www.outskirtspress.com

ISBN: 978-1-9772-0137-9

Cover Photos © 2020 Heather Hudak. All rights reserved - used with permission.

Outskirts Press and the "OP" logo are trademarks belonging to Outskirts Press, Inc.

PRINTED IN THE UNITED STATES OF AMERICA

For Mama Ruth

## Author's Note

The content of this book is for general instruction only. Each person's physical, emotional, and spiritual condition is unique. The instruction in this book is not intended to replace or interrupt the reader's relationship with a physician or other professional. Please consult your doctor for matters pertaining to your specific health and diet.

# Table of Contents

Gratitude ................................................................................... i

Acknowledgments ................................................................ iii

Introduction ........................................................................... v

One: What I Learned about Food in Nutrition School ................ 1

    What You Eat Matters. A Lot.
        (Think Fresh, Local, Organic, Seasonal) ........................... 3

    The Conscientious Carnivore .................................................. 7

    Happy Chickens Make Tasty Eggs ........................................... 8

    Poultry ..................................................................................... 10

    Dairy ....................................................................................... 10

    Fish ......................................................................................... 11

    Meat ........................................................................................ 11

    Fat, Beautiful Fat! ................................................................... 12

    A Little History ....................................................................... 12

    A Little Chemistry .................................................................. 13

    Choosing Fats ......................................................................... 14

    Fat & Heat .............................................................................. 16

    Digesting Fats ......................................................................... 16

Hey Sugar, You're Sweet Enough Already! ............................. 16

Your Body on Sugar ........................................................ 17

Sneaky Sugar .................................................................. 17

Make a Better Choice ..................................................... 18

Yikes, Please Don't ........................................................ 20

Your Happy Hydrated Cells ............................................ 20

Bio-individuality: Eating for the One and Only You ........ 22

My Personal Health Struggle: Bio-individuality in Action ...... 24

Respect Your Fellow Human's Food Choices (Pretty Please) ... 26

Primary Food: Feed Your Hunger for Life ....................... 26

## Two: The Care & Feeding of Your One and Only Body ............. 29

Becoming Curious ......................................................... 31

So, Where Are You? ...................................................... 32

Sort Out Your Food Issues (and A Word on Detoxing) .......... 37

How It Works ................................................................ 39

It's Been 23 Days: You Feel Awesome—Now What? ...... 41

Rotate & Rethink ........................................................... 43

Foods Your Body Wants You to Know About
  (This Is Your Shopping List) ........................................ 44

Wellness Teas = Alkalizing + Health Promoting .............. 53

Clean Beauty - Where to Start? ..................................... 60

## Three: Movement Is a Gift ............................................... 65

Creating Your Mindful Movement Practice .................... 67

Intention Starters .......................................................... 70

The Questions ............................................................... 70

The Answers (the "Why" to the "What") ........................ 70

Putting It All Together: Create Your Intention ................ 71

Shift Your Mindset: Movement & Mantras............................ 72

Create Your Mantra................................................................ 75

Your Mantra in Action ............................................................ 77

Core Strength, Personal Transformation, and
    How to Not Pee Your Pants ............................................... 78

Consistency Counts. A Lot. ..................................................... 81

Our Issues Are in Our Tissues ................................................. 83

Fascia Release.......................................................................... 84

## Four: What Is This Woo-Woo Stuff?
## (The Part Where I Talk about Your Chakras) ............................ 87

Are You Breathing, Honey? .................................................... 87

Your Spirit's Unfinished Business............................................ 88

You're in Your Feelings & Some of Them Suck—Now What? ...... 89

The Part Where I Talk about Your Chakras ........................... 89

What Is This Woo-Woo Stuff?................................................ 90

How I Use Energy Medicine (and How *You* Can Too!) .......... 92

Your (Brief) Energy Anatomy Lesson ..................................... 97

Qigong: Developing Energy Awareness ................................ 102

Chakras + Crystals ............................................................... 104

## Five: Cultivating Pleasure
## (The Part Where I Talk about Orgasms) ................................. 111

Your Brain on Pleasure: Yes, Please! ..................................... 112

Your Brain on Stress: Fight. Flight. Freeze. .......................... 113

Phew, That's Over! ............................................................... 114

Shake That Shit Off (Or, What My Dog Already Knows) .... 115

Don't Believe Everything You Think.................................... 116

Emotional Freedom Technique (EFT) Tapping.................... 119

Your Brain on Tapping ......................................................... 122

Like Riding a Bike .................................................................. 122
Tapping Your Truth................................................................ 123
8 Steps + 8 Points: Tapping Quick Start ................................ 124
Tapping Target: Your Limiting Belief..................................... 136
Peeling the Onion .................................................................. 139
Additional Tapping Resources ............................................... 140
The Pleasure List.................................................................... 141
What Brings *You* Pleasure? .................................................... 141
Finally, the Orgasm Part!....................................................... 143
#IAmNotAshamed ................................................................ 144
My Experience of Healing (Or, The Things I Wish I Knew) .... 144
#MeToo .................................................................................. 146
Transforming Shame into Love.............................................. 147
Honoring Your Lady Bits: Grab a Hand Mirror (Yes, Really).....148
What *Exactly* Am I Looking At? ............................................. 149
Crystals + Chakras + Self-Pleasure (Oh My!) ........................ 152
I Have Reflexology Points *Where?*........................................... 153
*Your* Jade Egg: Purchasing, Preparing, Practicing ................... 154
Practicing Pleasure ................................................................. 157
Sacred Yoni Bath .................................................................... 159
The Jade Egg & Magical Thinking ........................................ 160
Follow Your VPA ................................................................... 161

**Six: Love Yourself Up: Beauty Rituals from Head to Toe! ........ 163**
A Fancy Lady in a Modern World ......................................... 164
Love the Skin You're In ......................................................... 168
Beauty Rituals from Head to Toe: You Glow, Girl!................ 169

Beauty Secrets from Head to Toe:
  That Pretty Head of Yours ................................................ 179
Beauty Secrets from Head to Toe: Your Pearly Whites .......... 182
Beauty Secrets from Head to Toe:
  Your Perfectly Imperfect Breasts ...................................... 185
Beauty Rituals from Head to Toe: Your Lovely Lady Bits ..... 188
Upgrade Your Feminine Hygiene ............................................ 189
Your Feminine Essence: Clues to Health ................................. 189
Beauty Rituals from Head to Toe: Heavenly Hands +
  Fabulous Feet ..................................................................... 192
Beauty Secrets from Head to Toe: The Naked Truth ............ 195
Cellulite, Stretch Marks & Jiggly Bits ..................................... 195
Sing Your Soul Song ................................................................ 200
Mud Pie Magic ......................................................................... 201

**Seven: *Your* Path to Vibrant Health & Radiant Beauty** ............ 205
Creating Your Intention ......................................................... 205
It Starts With You, but You Don't Have to Go It Alone ....... 207
Health Coaching: What It Is + Why You Want It ................. 208
Functional Medicine: Health Care vs. Sick Care .................... 209
Chiropractic: Mind-Body Adjustment .................................... 210
Holistic Dentistry: Whole Body Health .................................. 211
Energy Medicine: Pick Your Woo Woo .................................. 212
Therapy: Keep an Open Mind ................................................ 212
Feed Your Mind. Mind Your Feed. ........................................ 214
Closing Meditation: Planting Seeds of Change ..................... 215

**Inspiration & Recommended Reading** ..................................... 217

**About the Author** ...................................................................... 221

# Gratitude

*"Holding space for someone is incredibly profound. When you hold space for someone, you bring your entire presence to them. You walk along with them without judgment, sharing their journey to an unknown destination. Yet you're completely willing to end up wherever they need to go. You give your heart, let go of control, and offer unconditional support. And when you do, both of you heal, grow and transform."*

— Lynn Hauka, Meditation Coach

**To my family:** My Parson, Smith, Harlow, Hudak and Hippie Friends Family—through you I continue to learn about the nature of family, forgiveness, hope, and love. My sisters Juliette Dannucci and Megan Gage, and soul sisters Andrea Land, Kelly Mulherron and Jennifer O'Hara, for keeping the promises of friendship whispered in our youth—you are my touchstones.

**To the boy I met when I was 10:** It was summer and I was sitting on the lawn outside Grandma Kay's house, squinting towards the sun to greet our mutual friend. I see you. Straddling your bike, hair a mess of curls and sunrays, eyes that pierce my soul with the sharp knowing of kindred spirits. Decades later, you say "jump with me" and I do (I always will).

**To my wellness team:** Ana E. Noles, PsyD, Jonathan Gavzer, LAc (aka my Functional Medicine Man), Dan Abels, LAc, and Jacalyn G. Buettner, DC, —your steady presence in my life reminds me that I am never alone on my healing path. You inspire me to live into wellness.

**To the IIN community:** Joshua Rosenthal, your vision of improving the world's health and happiness one health coach at a time inspired me to not only transform my own health, but the health of my family, friends and clients – your ripple effect in action! I am in deep gratitude to the teachers, fellow IIN coaches, and the Launch Your Dream Book course for supporting me in sharing my wellness journey.

**To the space holders:** Natalie Zee Drieu for editing these pages, bringing the cover to life, and endlessly supporting my creative endeavors. Your belief in me made writing this book possible. Wendy K. Yalom for encouraging me to speak my truth, shining a light on my path, and capturing my journey with your heart-shaped lens. Meg Messina for allowing me to witness your healing journey as you captured mine. Rosalyn Fay for holding my heart and inspiring me to heal the parts of myself that allowed me to write this book. Shelley Constantini and Darcy Hunt for your inspiration, encouragement, and (amazing) pro tips. Thank you for holding space for me, always.

**To the teachers + truth tellers + wise women:** Alexandra Jamieson, the work you do in the world, from your books and podcast to your social activism and art, has both supported me on my healing journey and modeled what it truly means to show up fully expressed in your work and in your life. The work you've done with me personally is the perfect combination of comfort zone pushing, empowering and magical. LiYana Silver, our chance meeting years ago was an "I'll have what she's having" moment that got me curious, led me to the path of Feminine Genius, and inspired me to turn toward my turn-on. Your Deep End community is the sacred space my heart has been longing for. Erin Stutland, your Say It Sweat It Get It Challenge found me in divine timing. Soul Strolling with your sweet voice in my ear holes has seen me through tricky times and created miracles in my life. Dr. Leslie Carr, your steady support of both my work and healing path is a beacon of hope, encouraging me to honor my own pace and each step of the journey. Jennifer Brinn, Karen Salinger and Sarah Tomlinson, my high vibe tribe - your wisdom and spiritual guidance make my soul sing.

**To the one and only *you*:** It is my great honor to share my story with you.

# Acknowledgments

**To my editors and publishing team:** Natalie Zee Drieu, Ruth Ann Parson, Brighid Ryan, and Outskirts Press

**Photographers:** Meg Messina and Wendy K. Yalom

**Hair & makeup stylists:** Cirilo De Jesus and Melissa Hoffman

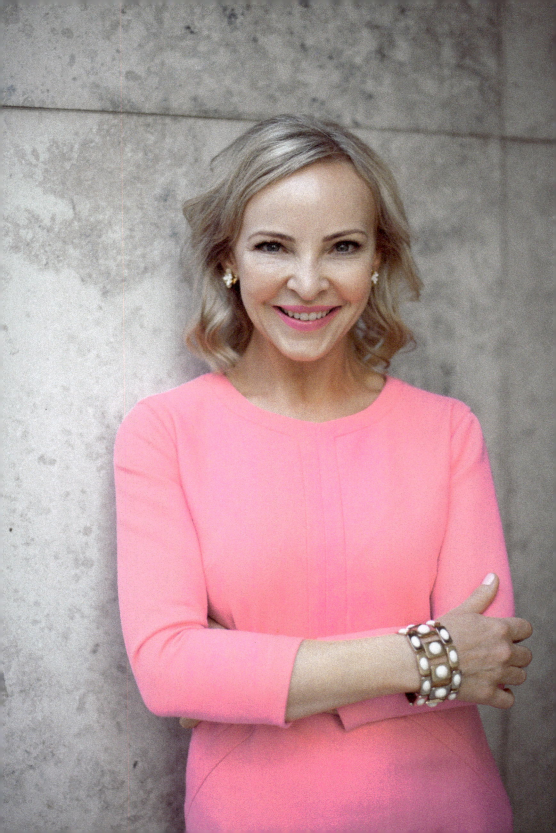

# Introduction

*"The dark night of the soul is a journey into light, a journey from your darkness into the strength and hidden resources of your soul."*
— Caroline Myss

The writing of this book unexpectedly coincided with a time in my life filled with difficult transitions, family health crises, and a lot of uncertainty (think Dark Night of the Soul). I started out wanting to share my story with you. The story of how my journey through complex life struggles, coupled with an unrelenting call from my soul to survive, mixed with an insatiable curiosity about the nature of wellness and beauty, led me to my life's work. *That* story starts like this:

I was ten years old when I overheard our family doctor tell my Grandma Kay, "Heather isn't just chubby anymore, she's fat." I got home that day and immediately went on the popular "crash diet" of the time - hard-boiled eggs, cottage cheese and grapefruit. That day in Dr. Greene's office marked the beginning of my struggle with disordered eating and negative self-image—a struggle that spanned decades, and threatened my physical, mental, and spiritual well-being. By the time I was a teenager I found myself stuck in a continuous cycle of dieting, binging, and purging. Most of my thoughts revolved around counting calories, planning my next workout, and readying myself to step into the ideal version of my life I was certain existed beyond the exhausting madness of my eating disorder. Being ready wouldn't happen until I hit the magic number on the scale, but the tricky thing was, as I stood there on the scale with this magic number starting back at me, my life still looked the same. A familiar sense of panic would set it - a panic only soothed by the repetition of starting the cycle all over again.

As the years passed, I continued to struggle, but I also started to heal. I began to recognize the thought patterns that led to my disordered eating. More and more time would pass between bouts of bulimia or anorexia. I became curious about my compulsive behavior, and when I found myself repeating old patterns, I would step back for a moment and ask myself what in my life needed attention. I saw the act of binging as a reenactment of "stuffing" my feelings deep inside my body; the act of purging was a welcome release both physically and emotionally. Taking that brief moment to ask myself the question "What in my life needs attention?" didn't necessarily break the cycle right then and there, but it got me closer every time. This time in my life taught me the meaning of progress, not perfection. It allowed me to be grateful for the times I was healthy, and to have compassion for myself when I was not. It was a lesson about finding my own balance and leaning in to health.

I was twenty-six when I got the phone call I had been preparing myself to receive since I was a child. My father's struggle with addiction, and a syringe of heroin, ended his forty-four years of life. It turns out being ready for that call wasn't a real thing. I am forever grateful to the many teachers along my path that held my hand, and my heart, along my healing journey. A decade after my father's passing, I was thriving in many aspects of my life. I enjoyed a healthier relationship with food, and while exercise remained an important aspect of my daily life, my movement practice was changing to reflect the deeper connection I felt with my body. I was sharing my life and love with my husband Jim—a childhood friend I met that very year I overheard Dr. Greene tell my grandmother I was fat. Then something unexpected happened; a devastating injury to my cervical spine left me in pain and unable to carry on with my life as I had been living it. Oscar Wilde's words "what seems to us as bitter trials are often blessings in disguise" would, in time, ring true.

I spent the next year exploring all manner of healing modalities in an effort to both avoid spinal surgery and manage my pain. To use one of my Mama Ruth's favorite phrases, "the gem in the shit" is that my struggle with an eating disorder sparked a passion for all things health and wellness early on. My natural curiosity and an open mind served me well. Alongside my prescribed physical therapy, I tried chiropractic, massage therapy, meditation, and various forms of Energy Medicine, including acupuncture, EFT Tapping, Qigong and Reiki. I also enrolled myself into the Institute for Integrative Nutrition's Health Coaching program to learn everything I could about the relationship between food and healing (I learned that and more). While I did eventually make the choice to undergo spinal surgery, the combination of therapies I was using had a healing impact far beyond the original intent. I developed a deep understanding of the saying "the issues are in the tissues" as layer by layer, I began to experience a deeper level of healing in my body, mind, and spirit.

Back to *this* story and what I want to tell you now: The experience of writing a wellness book while simultaneously experiencing a Dark Night of the Soul was a reminder of a simple truth that I sometimes find myself ignoring or trying to wish away. That truth is that there really is no end destination on your path to vibrant health. You don't get to "healed" and stay there. There is progress, not perfection. There are tools you learn along the way that you sometimes use and sometimes don't, but those tools will be there when you really need them (I promise). There are moments of profound clarity and joy and they are precious, but they can be fleeting. And that's okay.

I share my personal story with you not because it's unique; I share it with you because tragically, my story is not unique at all—only the small details belong to me and me alone. I share it because my story is your story, or your mother's story, or your best friend's story. It is the story of our society and the collective shame we feel about our bodies. It is the story of our families and our secrets and the way we learn to keep quiet. So quiet that your best friend doesn't know about your eating disorder. So quiet that you struggle with mental illness and you may even take your own life. By sharing my story with you, it is my hope that you will trust that you are not alone in your struggle, whatever your personal struggle may be. You possess within you an innate ability to heal, on all the levels you are. In these pages I will show you how listen to your body's own whisperings about what it truly needs to heal. In these pages, I invite you to become curious, to discover *your* own unique path to wellness, to live a life in line with your greatest vision for yourself. This *is* your "real life." Are you ready to live it like you mean it?

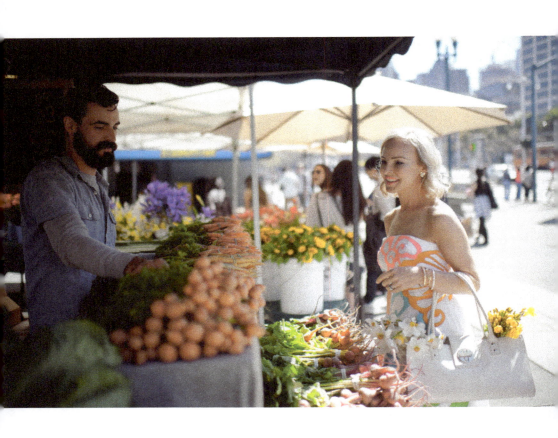

# Chapter One
# What I Learned about Food in Nutrition School

> *"Every decision we make about food is a vote for the kind of world we want to live in."*
> — Frances Moore Lappé, *Diet for a Small Planet*

**I developed some** interesting theories about food as a kid, most of them tied to my desire to be seen as "normal" to the world outside my family. My Mama Ruth was a young thing, raising me on her own with the dream of creating a better life for us. A better life included many things, not least of which was finding a way out of poverty, and an even quicker way out of the low-income housing in West Sonoma County, where we found ourselves living in the late 1970s. The path to this better life Mama Ruth envisioned was paved with long days working a job to make ends meet, and even longer nights of class and coursework to earn her master's in psychology. This path also made me part of a generation of latchkey kids—mine worn on a piece of green yarn tied around my neck.

The book *Diet for a Small Planet* turned Mama Ruth into an early adopter of the health food movement. It introduced her to the concept of food and planet mindfulness, and introduced me to a diet rich in vegetables, beans, and whole grains (I was not pleased). Money was tight in those days, but Mama Ruth was both creative and resourceful. These skills came in handy when confronted with the tricky task of making the food stamps last for a month of healthy eating. In place of bright-colored boxes of store-bought cereal were Mason jars filled with homemade granola. The walnuts from the tree in our backyard went into our granola recipe, and in the winter they made thrifty gifts for the holidays, packed in burlap and wrapped with a bow. The berries we picked on late summer days were preserved to spread on toast, the apples we harvested from a local orchard made into a sweet butter we mixed with homemade yogurt for a treat.

My idea of rebelling against Mama Ruth's hippie food was to get my hands on all of the "normal" food I could find. A look around my middle school cafeteria told me normal looked like Wonder Bread with American cheese and bologna, or a PB&J (Skippy was my favorite!) with grape jelly. Normal included something from Hostess, a bag of chips, and a fruit cocktail. My lunch? Not normal. Leftover brown rice topped with veggies and tofu made its way into recycled jars and called itself lunch. Other days, it might be a peanut butter sandwich like the other kids, only my version was served on sprouted grain bread and the peanut butter was made from actual peanuts (and nothing else) that we'd mixed in the machine at the health food store ourselves. Raw local honey stood in place for grape jelly, and no processed cheese or meat product ever found its way between slices of brown bread in my house. Open my sandwich and you'd find real white cheese and alfalfa sprouts that Mama Ruth sprouted herself in our kitchen window. There were no cupcakes or potato chips nestled in with the raw vegetables, trail mix, and (actual) fruit in my lunchbox, and nobody included me in the lunchtime tradsies game. Still, I didn't let that stand between me and my junk food fix. The latchkey kid thing sometimes had its perks, and in this case, some pretty sweet ones. Whenever I'd squirreled away enough change to make it worth the trip (and the afternoon school bus was out of sight), I'd walk the mile or so down our country road to the liquor store to buy as much candy as my pocket full of change could get me. Then I would eat it (all of it) on the slow walk back home.

Mama Ruth stocked our pantry with wholesome basics and prepared our meals with love. She also sometimes prepared them with tofu hot dogs, which is partly why I was so excited to eat dinner with the family next door on the nights she had class. Night classes for her meant frozen dinners and Kool-Aid for me! I would later understand that there was both a biochemical and emotional reason I was seriously stoked about the trifecta of sugar, fat, and salt served up at the neighbors' dinner table. These substances release opioids into our bloodstream, and when these chemicals bind with the receptors in our brain, we experience an intense sensation of pleasure (food scientists call this phenomenon the "bliss point"). Basically, I was getting high at the neighbors' house, and as much as I liked the novelty of eating what I then considered "normal" food, I missed eating dinner with my mom. Along with the "bliss point" of processed, chemicalized food, dinners with the family next door served up a good dose of emotional comfort for me.

## What You Eat Matters. A Lot.
## (Think Fresh, Local, Organic, Seasonal)

> *"The food you eat can either be the safest and most powerful form of medicine or the slowest form of poison."*
> — Ann Wigmore

While I may not have always embraced Mama Ruth's "hippie food," I am grateful that despite the obstacles (and my sweet tooth), she tried her darnedest to nourish my growing body and provide the foundational support of real, whole foods forming the basis of my meals growing up. While there are a lot of different perspectives on the ideal diet for humans, one thing every healthy dietary paradigm shares is an emphasis on whole foods. So, what is whole food? Whole foods are found in nature and made of one ingredient. Vegetables,

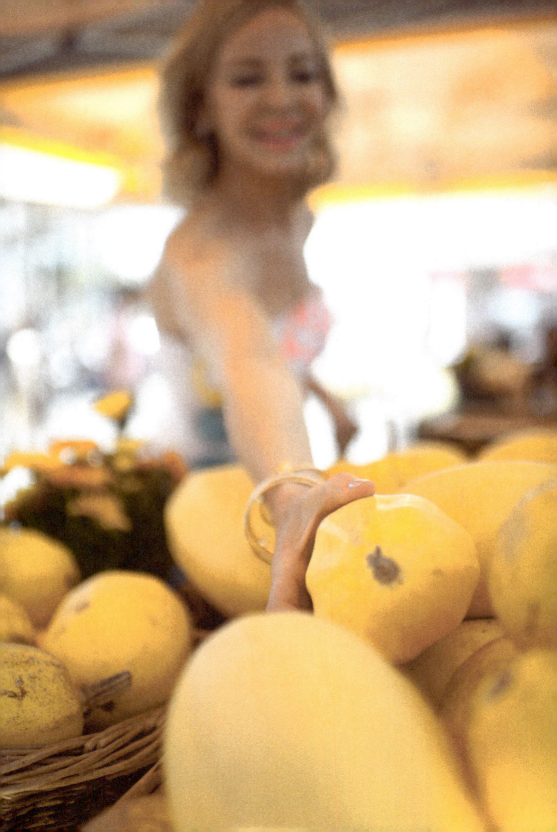

fruit, meat, fish, dairy, eggs, grains, legumes, nuts, and seeds are all examples of real, whole foods. On the other hand, processed foods contain all sorts of ingredients the body doesn't recognize, leading to inflammation and a weakened immune system. Inflammation in the body is at the core of many chronic diseases, lack of energy, and other so-called "age-related" conditions. Things like refined sugar, artificial sweeteners, processed vegetable oils, and artificial colors or flavors wreak havoc on your body (they do a number on your mind and spirit, too!).

When we educate ourselves about where our food comes from, we can better appreciate the importance of eating real, whole food. A regular trip to the farmers market is one of the best ways to do this! Meeting and talking to farmers and food artisans is a great opportunity to learn more about how and where food is produced. At the farmers market, you can find meats, cheeses, and eggs from animals that have been raised without hormones or antibiotics, that have grazed on green grass and eaten natural diets. Want to eat the yummiest produce ever? Choose vegetables and fruits harvested locally. The chemical composition of food changes radically a few hours after harvest, simply because it's been cut off from its food and water supply. With very little transportation time to the market, local produce will be at its peak in flavor! Not only will the food be tasty, the rich color of recently harvested produce indicates that more of the vital nutrients are present. Most farmers who sell their food locally don't artificially treat crops to withstand shipping and extend their shelf life. Buying locally supports your community, supports your health, and supports the intention of conserving global resources. By waiting for produce to be available locally only during certain windows of time, our eating has a cyclical feeling, keeping us in tune with the season. Keeping in tune with the season keeps us in tune with nature and with our bodies.

Large-scale farming works against the natural cycles of the earth, relying on chemicals to produce a larger yield. This process has depleted much of the world's soil of its vital minerals and nutrients. The resulting foods are not only deficient in nutrients, but they are also full of pollutants and agrochemicals. Pesticides, which are present in most commercial produce, must be processed by our immune systems and have been shown to cause cancer, as well as liver, kidney, and blood diseases. In addition, as pesticides build up in our tissues, our immune systems become more and more compromised, allowing other carcinogens and pathogens to affect our health. In contrast, organic farming works with the land. Crops are rotated from year to year to allow the soil to retain its nutrients between growing cycles. Animals graze in different areas each season to let grasses recover and replenish. Farmers feed the soil with compost, rather than using artificial fertilizing methods. Buying organic products is a form of voting. Your organic purchase says that you support the growers and manufacturers who are producing food without the use of synthetic fertilizers, insecticides, herbicides, or pesticides that pollute your body and our world.

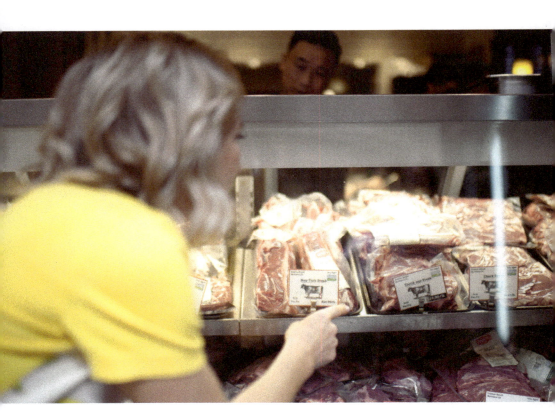

# The Conscientious Carnivore

> *"To get an idea of the conditions under which supermarket meat is raised, imagine if you were forced to eat Twinkies out of your own toilet ... it is the meat we eat from the hormone and disease-riddled commercially farmed animals that is making us sick, not the meat from animals that live and eat as nature intended."*
> — Kevin Gianni, author of *Kale and Coffee: A Renegade's Guide to Health, Happiness & Longevity*

I grew up vegetarian and I can't think of anybody who loves their veggies as much as I do (I find ways to include them at every meal), but my body is at its best when I also include animal protein. For me, finding high-quality, respectfully produced meat, poultry, fish, eggs, and dairy is one of my nonnegotiables. I don't want to support the inhumane, unhealthy processing plants where animals are treated as simply "product," so understanding where my food comes from is a priority for me. When selecting eggs, fish, birds, or animals, it is best if they have had access to their natural diet and have not been given antibiotics or hormones. Remember, you are what *they* eat. Speaking of eating, the sacred tradition of honoring the animal for its ultimate sacrifice by making use of all its parts is a wonderful way to align yourself with the principles of a conscientious carnivore. Finding a local butcher who uses the fat to make lard, the bones to make a nutritious stock, scrap pieces for sausage, and who sells the heart, liver, intestines, and other edible parts, is the perfect start! Treat the planet's animals well and eat with awareness of your food's impact on the whole. The choices you make when buying food have effects more far-reaching than their effect on your body and well-being. Here's a brief overview of what to look for!

# Happy Chickens Make Tasty Eggs

> *"A happy chicken is up with the dawn, lays an egg in the late morning, and when the farmer opens the little chicken house door, she heads outside to hunt for insects in the grass ... At dusk, the hen goes inside on her own, safe from predators, to her dinner of grain and oyster shell. That's how our chickens live at the farm."*
>
> — Nina Planck, author of *Real Food*

The natural diet for a chicken is bugs, worms, some grains, seeds, and greens. When birds eat this food, they produce incredible eggs! The yolks are golden orange and naturally rich in omega-3 fatty acids. Speaking of yolks, eat them for goodness' sakes! Contrary to popular belief, the cholesterol in the food you eat has virtually no impact on the cholesterol level of your blood. Blame sugar and processed carbs for the production of "bad" cholesterol in your body, not eggs. So, unless you have a food sensitivity (I'll help you sort that out in the next chapter), eat your eggs and eat them whole. No more egg white omelets! When you choose your eggs, you definitely want to avoid eggs from chickens that are treated poorly, fed antibiotics, and eat GMO feed; it's bad karma at best, so don't risk it.

Local, pasture-raised organic eggs are your best bet. Though the terms "cage free" or "free range" may sound appealing, it simply means that there are no cages in the chicken house and/or that the birds have access to the outside. "Pastured" is a relatively new term coined to explain the regimen of keeping birds in a moveable enclosure with nests and roosts that are moved once or twice daily to a new piece of grass, where chickens get at least 20 percent of their diet from foraging and eating insects. These are probably the highest-quality eggs you can purchase. You can find pastured eggs at a local farmers market or if you're lucky, you might have a friend with chickens like I do!

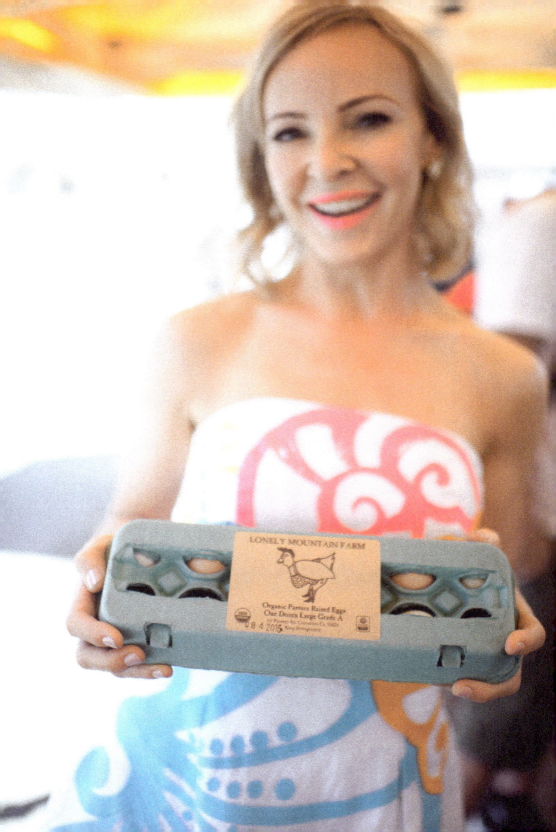

## Poultry

The term "organic" on poultry lets us know that the birds are fed organic feed, are not administered any antibiotics, and no irradiation or genetic modification has taken place. Raised under conditions that provide for exercise, access to the outdoors, and freedom of movement, organic is a good choice and labeling claims are verified by third-party inspectors. "Free range" or "free roaming" means that the poultry are not caged and the bird has had some access to the outdoors each day. The outdoor area must be 50 percent of the size of the barn area, and how long the bird or animal spends outside each day depends on the producer and the climate in which it is being raised. LocalHarvest.com is a terrific resource for a list of small-scale, local, and organic farms.

## Dairy

The choice to include or exclude dairy products can be confusing. Many cultures throughout history consumed fermented or cultured dairy foods such as yogurt, kefir, crème fresh, or aged cheeses in their diets. They did this because milk from other mammals can be a difficult food for humans to digest. Souring milk or adding live cultures breaks down both the milk sugar and milk protein, which are responsible for most digestive problems. Naturally cultured or fermented dairy products from soured milk not only add fat, protein, and minerals to the diet, but also friendly bacteria, which can help with the digestion of other foods. The practice of consuming homogenized, pasteurized milk is fairly recent and does contribute to health problems for some people. These same people often do quite well when they choose to consume full fat, raw dairy products. Reduced fat dairy products are no longer a whole food, as their nutritional composition has been altered, so picking whole fat is always the better option. Because antibiotics, hormones, and pesticides often get stored in the fat of the animal, which is then transferred to the milk, going organic is important if you choose to consume dairy. In his book *The New Health Rules*, Dr. Frank Lipman reminds us that it's a myth that radically reducing dairy in your diet will leave you calcium deficient. You can get all the calcium you need from dark green leafy vegetables like kale and spinach, without stressing your gut in the way that dairy can. He recommends thinking of dairy as a condiment, and I think that's a pretty sensible approach.

## Fish

Fish farming uses a variety of methods to grow or breed fish or shellfish in marine or fresh water. Fish farms currently provide one-third of all seafood. Fish farming can be done responsibly, but this is not always the case. Much of our farm-raised fish is genetically modified. Because of the sameness of the fish, disease spreads quickly and antibiotics must be used. The PBC levels are higher because the fish live in their own waste in a limited space. Farmed salmon are fed pellets to which coloring has been added to get the red color in the flesh. The best-quality fish are wild, line-caught fish. This means that the fish lived a normal life, ate a natural diet, and was caught in a sustained way. Look for fish with a shiny sheen, a fresh smell, and tight flesh (gaps in the flesh or yellowing are an indication of age—ick).

## Meat

Grazers (think cattle, sheep, and goats) are herbivores who do best when they are free to eat their natural diet of grass and other vegetation. Cows that are raised and finished on grass have more anti-inflammatory omega-3 fatty acids in their fat, making them a much healthier choice than their carnivorous (and sometimes cannibalistic) factory-farmed counterparts. It is not just the omega-3 fatty acid profile that makes grass-fed cows a better choice, it's … well, everything. In addition to being fed grain, which is not the natural diet of an herbivore, cattle are often fed less wholesome things like rendered poultry, pork, and even parts of other cattle deemed unfit for human consumption. Industrial cattle are treated with growth hormones to speed weight gain, and since their unnatural diet makes them sick, they are also fed antibiotics. Farmers who raise cows on pasture save money on feed, fertilizer, and vet bills. Let's support that! When choosing meat, go for "organic grass-fed" first or "certified humane raised and handled," which means that the cattle have sufficient space and shelter, access to fresh water at all times, and are not fed hormones or antibiotics. They must be treated and handled according to Humane Farm Animal standards, and these claims are verified by third-party inspectors.

## Fat, Beautiful Fat!

Want to be sexy *and* smart? Eat enough fat! The right fats are key to vibrant health and radiant beauty. Fat moisturizes and replenishes our skin, and keeps our hormone levels from declining. Healthy hormone levels help us maintain our youthfulness. If your body is deficient in high-quality fats, it's likely that you aren't producing hormones in adequate amounts. From the moment we are conceived, saturated fats become an important part of building our healthy body, playing a crucial role in brain and bone development in the womb. After birth, human milk supplies us with the saturated fat needed for our rapidly growing bodies. Fats make up 60 percent of the brain and are essential to brain function, including learning ability, memory retention, and emotional equilibrium. Saturated fats, like those found in ghee, raw butter, and grass-fed beef, also assist us in assimilating minerals—something many of us in the modern world are deficient in today.

## A Little History

In the early 1900s we consumed mostly saturated fats from butter, lard (rendered fat from pork), tallow (rendered fat from beef), palm oil, and coconut oil; and heart disease was rare. Then German chemist Wilhelm Normann patented the process to make hydrogenated vegetable oils, and by 1911, Procter & Gamble bought the rights, making Crisco commercially available for frying and baking. By 1950, heart disease became a leading cause of death in the U.S., and research indicated that vegetable oils were linked to this increase. In 1960 the American Heart Association issued a statement indicating that saturated fat correlated with heart disease, leading the vegetable-oil industry (corn, soybean, and peanut) to begin an attack on saturated fats, blaming meats, eggs, cheese, butter, and tropical oils (palm and coconut) as the heart disease culprits. From 1960 on, Americans began eating a "low-fat diet," including more refined, hydrogenated vegetable-based fats such as margarine made from corn, soybean, and safflower oils, contributing to epidemics of obesity, hormone imbalances, infertility, Alzheimer's, ADHD, and depression, as well as cancers, diabetes, and an increase in heart disease.

## A Little Chemistry

All fats consist of individual fatty acids made of hydrogen and carbon. Fatty acids may be saturated, monounsaturated, or polyunsaturated. These terms describe their chemical structure. All fatty acids are strings of carbon atoms encircled by hydrogen atoms. When every carbon atom bonds with a hydrogen atom, the fatty acid is saturated. If one pair of carbon atoms forms a bond, the fatty acid is monounsaturated. If two or more pairs of carbon atoms form a bond, the fatty acid is polyunsaturated. All the fats that we eat are a blend of saturated, monounsaturated, and polyunsaturated, and are identified by the predominant fatty acid. Butter is mostly saturated, olive oil is mostly monounsaturated, and corn oil is mostly polyunsaturated.

The body can manufacture some fats, while others, called essential, must be found in foods. The essential fats are polyunsaturated omega-3 and omega-6. These fats have equally important but opposite effects in the body. The ideal ratio is equal amounts of omega-3 and omega-6 fats, but the Standard American Diet (SAD) provides too few omega-3s and too much omega-6, which leads to inflammation, obesity, diabetes, heart disease, cancer, and depression.

Omega-3 fats include alpha-linoleic acid (ALA), docosahexaenoic acid (DHA), and eicosapentaenic acid (EPA). Flaxseed oil, grass-fed beef and butter, and pastured eggs all contain some omega-3 fats, but the ideal source is fish. The main omega-6 is linoleic acid (LA), found in grain and seed oils such as corn, safflower, and soybean oil. These sources of omega-6 are abundant in junk food and many Americans are getting way too much of it. On the other hand, gamma-linoleic acid (GLA) and conjugated linoleic acid (CLA) are two omega-6 fats that we should be eating more of. The best sources are borage, black currant seed, and evening primrose. GLA reduces inflammation, dilates blood vessels, reduces clotting, and aids in fat metabolism. CLA, which fights cancer and builds lean muscle, is found almost exclusively in grass-fed beef and grass-fed butter.

## Choosing Fats

> *"If you're trying to remember which fats are healthy, follow this rule: eat the foods we've eaten for thousands of years in their natural form. If you can't find the perfect version of a food—say 100% grass-fed beef—look for the next best thing. Any version of the traditional fats will be better for you than any version of the industrial fats. Those you must avoid like the proverbial Black Death."*
>
> — Nina Planck

I'm a huge fan of food writer and farmers market entrepreneur Nina Planck. Raised on her family's farm in Virginia and fed on simple real foods like raw milk and a lot of vegetables, Nina opened the first farmers markets in London in 1999. Her company, London Farmers' Markets, runs 18 year-round markets. Her books *Real Food: What to Eat and Why* and *Real Food for Mother and Baby* greatly influenced my own food philosophy and inspired me to do the majority of my food shopping at our local farmers market. This handy chart is adopted from *Real Food* and gives you some simple guidelines to follow when choosing traditional healthy fats over industrial fats:

**The Basics**

- All the traditional fats are healthy.
- The industrial diet contains too many omega-6 fats and too few omega-3 fats. This leads to obesity, diabetes, heart disease, cancer, and depression.
- Trans fats lower HDL and cause heart disease.
- With animal fats, the animal's diet matters for our own health.
- With vegetable oils, processing matters for our health.

**Traditional Animal Fats: Eat Up**

- Fat from grass-fed cattle, sheep, bison, and other game
- Butter and cream from grass-fed cows
- Lard from pastured pigs fed a natural diet
- Egg yolks from pastured chickens, ducks, and geese
- Fish oils (preferably wild), especially cod-liver oil

**Vegetable Oils: Eat Up**

- Cold-pressed, extra-virgin olive oil
- Cold-pressed, unrefined flaxseed oil
- Wet-milled, unrefined coconut oil
- Cold-pressed, unrefined macadamia nut oil
- Cold-pressed, unrefined walnut oil
- Cold-pressed, unrefined sesame oil

**Modern Industrial Fats: Avoid**

- All hydrogenated and partially hydrogenated oils, including lard and all vegetable oils

- Corn, safflower, sunflower, and soybean oils, especially when refined or heated

## Fat & Heat

The type of fat you choose to cook with matters. The more saturated a fat, the sturdier it is, because saturated bonds are stronger than unsaturated bonds. Unsaturated bonds are easily damaged or oxidized by heat, and oxidized fats can contribute to a whole host of things we don't want like cancer, heart disease, Alzheimer's and liver disease. So, what to cook with? For roasting and sautéing, butter from grass-fed cows, ghee, or coconut oil are all great choices.

## Digesting Fats

If you have difficulty digesting fats and oils, it's likely that your liver and/or gallbladder are congested. Symptoms of fat intolerance can include painful spasms in the large and small intestines, feeling tired just after eating, bloating, indigestion, belching, flatulence and/or nausea, upper-right abdominal discomfort, and hard stools. If you are experiencing any of these symptoms and suspect you are not digesting fats well, try testing one fat at a time and pay close attention to your body. Finding a good digestive enzyme can help your assimilation of fats, but it's also worthwhile to look for ways to support your liver and gallbladder.

## Hey Sugar, You're Sweet Enough Already!

William Dufty's book *Sugar Blues* was first published in 1975; and much to my dismay, Mama Ruth read it. Cover to cover. Not that she allowed much sugar into the house prior to being empowered with the knowledge that sugar was undermining her intention of growing me up healthy, but now it was full out banned. Needless to say, I was pretty bummed about our sugar-free household (and okay, I snuck candy any chance I got), but now I admit the wisdom of her decision. If one of your goals is vibrant health and radiant beauty, then sugar is best kept to a minimum. Even better, ditch the white stuff (even if it's brown or labeled "raw") and explore some healthier options.

## Your Body on Sugar

Sugar raises your risk of heart disease, cancer, diabetes, and Alzheimer's. Not to mention the number it does on your skin (premature wrinkles—no thanks!). Glucose is the sugar that gets processed in our gut during digestion and can ultimately be used by every cell in our body. Fructose bypasses the gut completely and goes straight to our livers. Some of it gets stored as glycogen, but some of it gets turned into triglycerides (a fancy term for fats). The Standard American Diet (SAD) is loaded with sugars, including fructose, which in its purest form is 70% sweeter than table sugar, making it even more addictive. Eating too much food with fructose leads to a slower metabolism and is correlated to a number of chronic diseases. Fructose can also cause leptin resistance, which is the hormone that tells your body whether you are hungry or full. Foods high in sugar trigger the reward centers in the brain, alter the biochemical pathways in our brain, and mess with our dopamine receptors. In order for us to get the next dopamine spike, we need a greater dose of sugar. Sugar is basically crack.

## Sneaky Sugar

Just as sugar likes to hide in processed foods like bread, salty snacks, and yogurt, it also likes to disguise itself with different names. Sneaky sugar! One of the easiest ways to recognize sugar on a food label is by recognizing the –ose suffix. When you find words that end in –ose, there is a good chance it's sugar (Sucrose, Maltose, Dextrose, Glucose, Galactose, Lactose, High Fructose corn syrup, Glucose solids).

# Make a Better Choice

If you have a sweet tooth and you're making a concerted effort to get yourself off sugar, the supplement glutamine can help. Glutamine is an amino acid that tricks your body into thinking it's getting sugar. Sweet, right?! Another trick we learned in nutrition school was to incorporate more sweet vegetables, like roasted beets and sweet potatoes, into your daily diet. Eating is a source of pleasure and, as you will read later in this book, pleasure is a vital ingredient in your wellness plan. If you like the sweet stuff, give yourself permission to savor your favorite desserts on occasion. And while doing so, I encourage you to use moderation, explore natural, healthier options, and listen to your body. One of the things your body might be telling you is that you are sweet enough already.

**Good Alternatives:**

- **Coconut Sugar:** Coconut sugar is the boiled and dehydrated sap of the coconut palm. This form of sugar does offer some trace nutrients and may have less of a dramatic impact on your blood sugar than other types of sweeteners.
- **Blackstrap Molasses:** This was a staple in my Mama Ruth's kitchen when I was growing up and I still love its taste, although I admit it isn't for everyone. Organic blackstrap molasses is one of the most nutritious sweeteners derived from sugar cane or sugar beet, and is made by a process of clarifying and blending the extracted juices. The longer the juice is boiled, the less sweet, more nutritious, and darker the product is. It's a good source of iron, which is one of the reasons my Chinese herbalist has me take the occasional spoonful.
- **Date Sugar:** If you like the taste of dates, date sugar consists of finely ground, dehydrated dates and can be used as a direct replacement for sugar in its granulated form. It's not the best option for certain baked goods, though, as it can clump and it doesn't melt.

- **Raw Honey:** This is one of my favorite sweeteners and you'll learn more about its health and beauty benefits later in this book! Honey is one of the oldest natural sweeteners and, depending on the plant source, can have a range of flavors from dark and strongly flavored, to light and mild in taste.
- **Maple Syrup & Sugar:** Maple syrup is made from boiled-down maple tree sap and contains many minerals. It adds a pleasant flavor to foods (I love it in Sacred chocolates!) and is great for baking. Be sure to buy organic 100% maple syrup and not maple-flavored corn syrup (yuck). Also, Grade B is stronger in flavor and said to have more minerals than Grade A. Maple sugar is created when the sap of the sugar maple is boiled for longer than is needed to create maple syrup. Once most of the water is evaporated, all that is left is the solid sugar. Maple sugar is as sweet as standard granulated sugar, but much less refined.
- **Stevia:** This leafy herb has been used for centuries by native South Americans, and the extract from stevia is 100 to 300 times sweeter than white sugar. It can be used in cooking, baking, and beverages, but does not affect blood sugar levels and has zero calories. Stevia is available in a powder or liquid form. Be sure to purchase the green or brown liquids or powders, because the white and clear versions are highly refined.
- **Lucuma:** Lucuma has been used for centuries in South America for its medicinal properties. Made from the subtropical fruit of the Pouteria lucuma tree, the taste is subtly maple-like. In addition to satisfying your sweet tooth without making your blood sugar levels soar, lucuma has health and beauty benefits that make it a really great choice. Rutgers University conducted a study that evaluated the anti-inflammatory effects of lucuma on wound closure and skin aging that determined the extract of the fruit may have anti-inflammatory, anti-aging, and skin-repair effects on human skin.

## Yikes, Please Don't

Artificial sweeteners lack calories and are advertised as a healthy alternative to high-fructose corn syrup and sugar. However, studies have shown that consuming artificial sweeteners such as saccharin (Sweet'N Low), sucralose (Splenda) or aspartame (Equal and NutraSweet) might make you gain weight faster than if you were consuming regular sugar. Artificial sweeteners slow your metabolism and ultimately trigger you to eat more. The three main ingredients in artificial sweeteners—aspartame, saccharin, and acesulfame potassium—have all been linked to cancer as well as Alzheimer's, autism, chronic fatigue syndrome, lupus, multiple sclerosis, and Parkinson's disease. Yikes, please don't!

## Your Happy Hydrated Cells

Your body loves water! Water carries nutrients to every single one of your cells, flushes toxins, regulates body temperature, and protects your joints and organs. On the flip side, dehydration can have adverse health effects like low blood pressure, headache, fatigue, disorientation, and food cravings (especially for sweets). The guidance on how much water we need to drink varies for each person contingent on a number of factors, but a simple strategy for determining how much water you need for optimum hydration is to become more conscious of how you are feeling and be able to discern the signals of dehydration. Our bodies are very intuitive and well equipped to help us determine the right amount of hydration. One of the ways it does this is by giving us clues and hoping we catch on.

**You Have Happy Hydrated Cells:**

- You rarely feel thirsty, but keep a glass of water handy to sip throughout the day.
- Your girlfriends always comment on your glowy skin and want to know your secret.

- You can stand naked in a dressing room with fluorescent lighting and still have to squint to see your cellulite.
- You poop like a rock star.
- Your pee runs clear, light yellow, or straw color (note: intensely colored foods, some medications, and B vitamins can make your urine dark, even if you are hydrated).
- You continuously produce sweat during heavy physical exertion and notice an overall higher-quality athletic performance.
- The app on your smart scale tells you so.

**Your Cells Are Craving Water:**

- You are thirsty. Like really, really thirsty.
- Your girlfriends are too polite to say anything, but you have bad breath.
- You stand naked in a dressing room with fluorescent lighting and make yourself a note to buy a loofah and a super good moisturizer.
- Your poop (if you even have any) resembles rabbit pellets.
- Your pee runs dark and is kinda smelly.
- You don't sweat much, even when you work out strenuously, which you rarely do because you can't seem to find the energy.
- The app on your smart scale tells you so.

Being well hydrated can be a bit of a challenge, even if we are drinking that "8 glasses a day" we've heard so much about. The problem is, as we age, our cells and connective tissue become damaged and not as efficient at holding water as they once were. So, all the water we are diligently downing that should end up in our cells and connective tissues ends up in the spaces between (puffy eyes, anyone?). Find yourself a pure water source and then work towards repairing your cells and connective tissue by consuming real whole foods, including the healthy fats I talked about in the first chapter (go ahead and reread that).

Adding a few pinches of Celtic Grey Mineral Sea Salt or Himalayan Pink Salt is a great way to support your happy, hydrated cells. This is referred to as "charging" your water. "Charging water" means giving a life-pattern or structure to the water at a microscopic level. These salts contain more than eighty different minerals, unlike table salt and most "kiln-dried" sea salts that have had their minerals oxidized away through heating. Squeezing fruit juices or placing leaves of plants into water is another great way to charge your water. The bonus? You will be rewarded with skin that glows, less cellulite, improved memory, and better poop! All these wonderful things because your cells are happy and hydrated ... cheers!

## Bio-individuality: Eating for the One and Only You

*"Trust your own instinct. Your mistakes might as well be your own, instead of someone else's."*
— Billy Wilder

Clients often come to me with the question, "What should I eat?" My answer is that I don't know, but I'm here to support them in finding out. This can be disappointing for the person looking for a quick fix or the lowdown on the latest dietary craze, but I can promise you that if you do the work to discover what foods work best for you, your life will change for the better. Discovering which foods work best in your one and only body (within the organic, whole foods category, of course!) is key. This requires an open mind, as well as some experimentation and personal testing. Getting to know your own body is an essential first step.

When I studied at the Institute for Integrative Nutrition (IIN), we had the amazing opportunity to explore more than 100 different dietary theories taught by world-class educators who are leading physicians, researchers, doctors, and nutrition experts at the forefront of the health and wellness movement. With all this information available to us, figuring out what to eat to be our most vital, healthy selves should have been a piece of (organic, gluten-free, naturally sweetened) cake. But the most common experience amongst my fellow students was that most of us, myself included, were following whatever dietary theory the current guest instructor was lecturing about. If it was David Wolfe (hello, raw cacao!), we were all experimenting with Superfoods; when IIN founder Joshua Rosenthal introduced us to the teachings of Michio Kushi, we leaned toward a macrobiotic lifestyle. Each speaker presented compelling information delivered with such enthusiasm, it was super easy to hop on board and claim the dietary theory of the week as our own. Then we were introduced to one of the most important concepts we learned about in nutrition school—bio-individuality; or "one person's food is another person's poison." Bio-individuality tells us that no one way of eating works perfectly for everyone. Differences in anatomy, metabolism, body composition, and cell structure all influence your overall health and the foods that work best for you. Bio-individuality is why some people do better eating more animal protein, while others do better eating less; and still others find that a vegetarian or vegan diet is best for them. The food that is ideal for you may not work at all for your best friend. Similarly, no one way of eating will work perfectly for you all the time.

In the following chapter you will have an opportunity to experiment with what foods work well for your body, but a very simple way of doing this is to keep a food journal for a week. Take note of what you ate and how that particular food made you feel both immediately after eating, and a few hours later. Did you feel satisfied and energized, or did you feel heavy and tired? Did you have an initial boost of energy only to find that energy plummeting shortly afterward? Did you feel satisfied at the end of your meal, but ravenous shortly after? The answers you discover are clues to your own bio-individuality. This approach to eating will naturally guide you to the foods that best support you for this time in your life.

# My Personal Health Struggle: Bio-individuality in Action

I have always been an active person. A typical day in my life includes a walk with our dog Gello, followed by more "formal" exercise (Yoga, Pilates, TRX, or the Tracy Anderson Method, depending on the day). Having lived in both San Francisco and Manhattan (two fantastic walking cities) most of my adult life, I'm also in the habit of running many of my errands by foot. According to the app on my iPhone, I easily cover around 7 miles a day just tending to the basics of my life. When I found myself needing to rest partway through Gello's morning walk to steady myself from frequent bouts of weakness, dizziness, shortness of breath, and heart palpitations, I knew it was time to speak with a professional about my symptoms. On particularly bad days, I needed to rest during simple household chores, like making my bed. I struggled with fertility issues, including several early miscarriages, and often found myself waking up in the night covered in sweat (a telltale sign of hormonal imbalance). More often than not, I was plagued by a vague but very real sense of anxiety or "impending doom," and my muscles ached in a way that felt unrelated to my movement practice. Most alarmingly, I'd begun experiencing what felt like electric shocks, often in my face and chest. These shocks tended to strike without warning, and left me feeling even more anxious about the mounting symptoms I was experiencing in my body.

It was 2010 and here I was, newly certified as an Integrative Nutrition Health Coach, and I had never felt worse in my life. I was confused, frustrated, and frankly a bit scared. I felt like I was doing everything right, but this vibrant health I was seeking felt further and further out of reach. My Primary Care Physician (PCP) ran a full blood panel, an EKG, and pulmonary function tests. When the results came back, I braced myself for difficult news only to be advised that I was in perfect health. Perfect health—how could that be?! The vision I held for myself of "perfect health" certainly didn't include heart palpitations or not being able to change my sheets without taking a break to steady myself. While I was relieved to know I wasn't facing a devastating diagnosis, I still found myself in need of answers.

I was familiar with the term *functional medicine* from nutrition school, and had been meaning to find one in my community, so I used this opportunity to do some research. Looking back, this step was the single most important thing I've done towards my health. Not only because I was able to finally get to the bottom of why I was experiencing these debilitating and sometimes frightening symptoms, but also because I felt empowered as a partner in my own health care for the first time in my life. This inspired me to take responsibility for both defining and creating my own vision of vibrant health and well-being. This was a paradigm shift.

Working with my Functional Medicine Practitioner (FMP), I began to understand the concept of bio-individuality on a personal level. My intellectual ideas about what foods "should" work in my body were in conflict with my bio-individual needs. I had been leaning towards a diet high in raw foods and light on animal products, and was combining this with regular detoxing and a strenuous workout regime. While this could be the ideal recipe for vibrant health during some phases of my life, during this particular time I was unknowingly struggling with chronic anemia, absorption issues, and depletion of my hypothalamic-pituitary-adrenal axis, the body's stress-regulating system. I also had unresolved emotional issues that needed tending to. Together, we worked on creating a plan that addressed not only my physical symptoms, but took into account my emotional and spiritual needs as well. This was not your typical "prescription" and there were no quick fixes here, although grass-fed beef sorted out my anemia pretty darn fast. Instead, I was supported on a path that would allow me to develop a new relationship with my body—a relationship that allowed me to tune in to both the subtle and not-so-subtle messages my body had been sending me about what it needed to heal. *Your* body has messages for you too.

## Respect Your Fellow Human's Food Choices (Pretty Please)

Bio-individuality tells us that the "perfect" diet doesn't exist, which allows each of us the opportunity for personal exploration. Every person is unique in terms of the foods they will thrive on. Your intellectual ideas about what to eat may be quite different from what your body knows to be true, or what is true for your friend, colleague, or relative. Being a compassionate human means respecting the food choices of others, even when their beliefs don't align with our own.

## Primary Food: Feed Your Hunger for Life

> *"Nutrition is everything you consume and everything you surround yourself with. It's the thoughts and feelings you ingest, the energy of the space you inhabit, and the interactions you have with others on a daily basis."*
> — Joshua Rosenthal, author of *The Power of Primary Food: Nourishment Beyond the Plate* and founder of the Institute for Integrative Nutrition

Joshua Rosenthal coined the term "primary food" to describe the many non-food "foods" that people need in order to feel happy, secure, and fulfilled. Through this concept, he expanded his teachings about nutrition to include more than the food we put into our mouths—nutrition is everything you consume and everything you surround yourself with. It's the thoughts and feelings you ingest, the energy of the space you inhabit, and the interactions you have with others on a daily basis. When a person's primary food is working well for them, making healthy choices around food is almost second nature. Your relationships, physical activity, self-care practices, career, and spirituality are all examples of primary food. When a person's primary food is suffering, all the green smoothies in the world won't magically bring about the balanced life they desire.

Sometimes a positive transformation can begin with making just one minor adjustment. Because health is integrative, each time you take action to improve your level of happiness in one area of your life, you'll create momentum that will flow into other areas of your life as well. We must be willing to look at the integrated whole of our lives and take meaningful action to bring about the change we seek. Throughout this book, we will do just that!

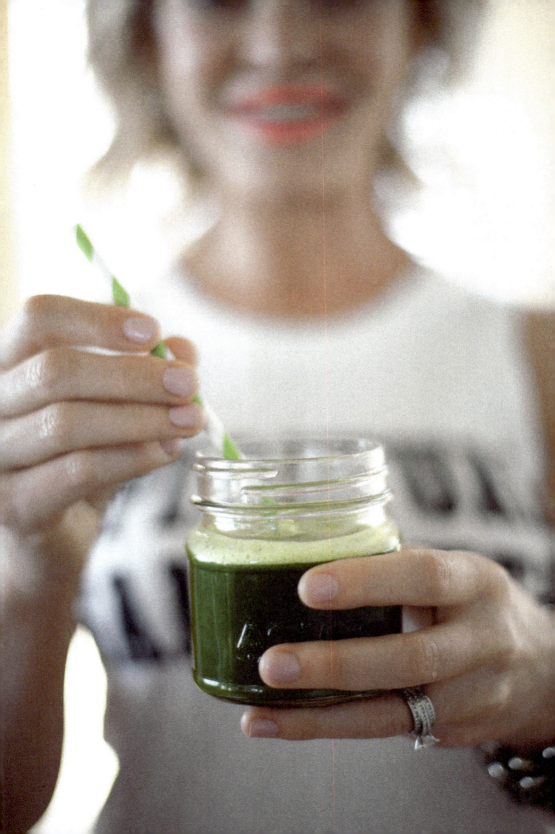

# Chapter Two
# The Care & Feeding of Your One and Only Body

*"I believe that a healthy person has the most important ingredients to their health built into their system. Our health is an expression of the ability to be self-regulating. When it's time to eat and when we've had enough, when it's time to rest and when to act, etc., are all senses that we are born with. Through our traumas, pathologies and stresses, these messages can get overlooked and eventually become disturbed enough so that we stop living according to them."*
— Jonathan Gavzer, LAc, Functional Medicine Practitioner

**I was ten** years old when I overheard our family doctor tell my Grandma Kay, "Heather isn't just chubby anymore, she's fat." I got home that day and immediately went on whatever "crash diet" was popular at the time (think hard-boiled eggs, cottage cheese, and grapefruit). That day in Dr. Greene's office marked the beginning of my struggle with disordered eating and negative self-image—a struggle that spanned decades, and threatened my physical, mental, and spiritual well-being. By the time I was a teenager I was in a continuous cycle of dieting, binging, and purging. Most of my thoughts revolved around counting calories, planning my next workout, and readying myself to step into the idealized version of my life I was certain existed beyond the exhausting madness of my eating disorder. Being ready wouldn't happen until I hit the magic number on the scale, but the tricky thing was, as I stood there on the scale with this magic number staring back at me, my life still looked the same. A familiar sense of panic would set in—a panic only soothed by the repetition of starting the cycle all over again.

We each have our own set of circumstances setting the stage for disordered behavior around food, and while Dr. Greene's words surely tapped into feelings of shame and underdeveloped self-worth, he didn't create those feelings. You certainly don't need a diagnosable eating disorder to have a complicated relationship with food. One of the lessons I learned over my decades-long struggle with disordered eating is that my body always did know how to heal. I always did have the choice to either listen to its messages or drown them out with whatever distraction felt safest to me in the moment. You have that choice too. The other lesson I learned was that change takes time. You likely already know this (or at least suspect it), and you might not be happy about it. Personally, I find comfort in that knowledge, because it allows me to step back and take a look at the big picture. The big picture of your health is that every positive action you take toward feeling your most vibrant, healthy self has an impact. You don't have to feel overwhelmed by the idea of making *all the changes* today. It kinda takes the pressure off, right? The other cool thing about change taking time is that it doesn't always take a *long* time for healthy changes to make a noticeable difference in your life.

In the first chapter you had an opportunity to explore the idea of primary vs. secondary food. Nutrition is everything you consume and everything you surround yourself with. It's the food you eat, the thoughts and feelings you ingest, the energy of the space you inhabit, and the interactions you have with others on a daily basis. Your relationships, physical activity, career, and spiritual practice are all examples of primary food. In this chapter, our focus is going to be on secondary food, which is what you put into your mouth (and onto your body) to nourish yourself … or not (we'll sort that out).

You can use food to feel the way you want to feel, look the way you want to look, and live the life you want to live. The goal is to become clearer on the connection between what you eat and how you feel. This knowledge will empower you to take responsibility for your own wellness.

Back to what I said about not all changes taking a long time to make a noticeable difference in your life. While there is certainly more than one way to achieve health, happiness, and beauty, there are changes you can begin making today that will not only bring about lasting wellness that you can both see and feel, but some of the benefits can be pretty immediate. A lifelong curiosity about all things health and wellness, coupled with my personal quest for healing, has given me the opportunity to test *a lot* of these methods. What I've found is that sorting out your food issues and reducing your toxic burden are two simple yet powerful ways to bring about positive change in a (relatively) short amount of time. In this chapter we're going to explore some creative ways you can reduce your toxic load, boost your body's own ability to detox, and discover which foods best support your one and only body.

## Becoming Curious

While I used to strongly identify with the clinical label of "eating disorder," I no longer do; but not for the reason you may think. While it's true that I no longer engage in the behavior that prompted that diagnosis, the reason I let go of that label is that I found the mindset of "having an eating disorder" did more to support my belief that something was wrong with me than support my intention to heal. I stopped identifying with "bulimic" or "anorexic" long before I stopped binging, purging, or restricting food; and in that subtle shift I found a freedom that allowed me to become curious about my behavior. As I became curious, self-judgment stepped aside for compassion, and healing followed. I believe that curiosity saved my life. What might happen in your life if you became curious?

As you do the work in this chapter, I invite you to set aside your own limiting beliefs about food and your body, whatever they may be. You can go ahead and replace them with the belief that your body is a miracle with amazing things to teach you! While embarking on change is awesome and exciting, it can also be kinda scary. Sometimes the truth of our lives can be so far out of alignment with what we envision for ourselves that we can get a little panicky. If you begin to feel overwhelmed at any point in this chapter, you can be reassured that positive transformation can begin with making just one minor adjustment. Take your time. Go Slow. You are right where you need to be.

## So, Where Are You?

This is an exercise to help you get in touch with how you feel in your body—right here, right now. This is *not* a starting point for beating yourself up about any habits you consider "bad." This is simply your chance to become curious about where you are, how you feel, and to consider how you might like to feel different. This is your opportunity to really check in with yourself, so even though you might have the urge to "clean up your act" as you go through this exercise today, I want to encourage you to go about your normal, everyday routine. Nobody is looking but you, so go ahead and grab your journal, and let's get started!

### *A Day in the Life of the One and Only You*

**Rise and Shine:**

- How do you feel when you first wake up—refreshed or snoozy?
- Does your mood and energy level vary day to day?
- How are you feeling right now?
- How would you like to feel?

**Everybody Eats:** Please take a moment to record what you ate and drank.

**Everybody Poops:** Please take a moment to record your bodily functions (and be specific).

**Your Body Loves to Move:** Please take a moment to record your physical activity.

## Midmorning:

- By now you've gone through your morning routine (unless you're still asleep); what did that look like for you?
- Did you make time for self-care?
- How do you feel right now?
- How would you like to feel?

**Everybody Eats:** Please take a moment to record what you ate and drank.

**Everybody Poops:** Please take a moment to record your bodily functions (and be specific).

**Your Body Loves to Move:** Please take a moment to record your physical activity.

## Noon:

- How did your morning routine make you feel?
- How did what you ate for breakfast make you feel?
- How are you feeling right now?
- How would you like to feel?

**Everybody Eats:** Please take a moment to record what you ate and drank.

**Everybody Poops:** Please take a moment to record your bodily functions (and be specific).

**Your Body Loves to Move:** Please take a moment to record your physical activity.

### Midafternoon:

- How did what you ate for lunch make you feel?
- How is your energy level?
- How do you feel right now?
- How would you like to feel?

**Everybody Eats:** Please take a moment to record what you ate and drank.

**Everybody Poops:** Please take a moment to record your bodily functions (and be specific).

**Your Body Loves to Move:** Please take a moment to record your physical activity.

### Evening:

- Who prepared your evening meal and who else is sitting around your table?
- What does your typical evening routine look like?
- How do you wind down at the end of the day?
- How do you feel right now?
- How would you like to feel?

**Everybody Eats:** Please take a moment to record what you ate and drank.

**Everybody Poops:** Please take a moment to record your bodily functions (and be specific).

**Your Body Loves to Move:** Please take a moment to record your physical activity.

**Bedtime:**

- What's your favorite bedtime ritual?
- Is it typically easy for you to fall asleep? How about staying asleep?
- How do you feel right now?
- How would you like to feel?

**Everybody Eats:** Please take a moment to record what you ate and drank.

**Everybody Poops:** Please take a moment to record your bodily functions (and be specific).

**Your Body Loves to Move:** Please take a moment to record your physical activity.

Now it's time to get curious! As you look over your answers to these questions, take note of when the way you were feeling wasn't how you wanted to feel. Perhaps you noticed that you didn't wake up feeling rested even though you'd had plenty of sleep. Maybe all my pestering you about your poop has you wondering if something might be slowing down your digestion. Or, maybe you didn't exercise because the food you ate didn't provide the energy to make good on your intention to move more. Maybe starting where you are looks like sorting out your food issues so you can finally figure out what in your diet is keeping you from looking and feeling your best, or maybe starting where you are looks like upgrading your lifestyle by making some simple changes to your everyday routine. Maybe it looks like both.

## *Becoming Curious: Where Should You Start?*

There are a number of reasons a person might not feel the way they want to feel. Sometimes it's a physical reason, sometimes it's an emotional or spiritual reason, but most often it's a combination of all three. While we will be exploring ways to find more balance in each of these areas throughout this book, experience has taught me that feeling better inside your body can make other seemingly pressing issues magically disappear! Obviously, this makes it the perfect place to start.

One way we can begin to feel better inside our body is to get curious about how we react to the foods we are consuming, particularly ones that may be "toxic triggers" for us. Toxic triggers are foods that cause indigestion, inflammation, bloating, fatigue, and a whole host of other unpleasant symptoms. If consumed over long periods of time, toxic triggers have the potential to cause major health challenges. The best method for discovering your own toxic triggers is to test them; and while the accuracy of food sensitivity tests is improving, testing through dietary change remains the gold standard. So, what exactly does this look like? Sorting out your food issues looks like removing potential toxic triggers by adhering to an elimination diet for a set period of time (23 days to be exact), and then reintroducing the potential triggers back into your diet in a way that allows you to really connect with how each food makes you feel.

Periodically eliminating specific foods is an amazing tool for self-discovery and a powerful act of self-care. If you suspect you are struggling with a hidden food allergy, or want to discover which foods make you look and feel your best, this is an awesome way to do that. That said, sorting out your food issues does come with some minor inconveniences (physical and emotional), especially in the beginning as you adjust to making changes in your diet. If you've been relying on coffee or sugar to get you through the day, or like to wind down in the evening with a glass (or two) of wine, you *will* go through a period of adjustment.

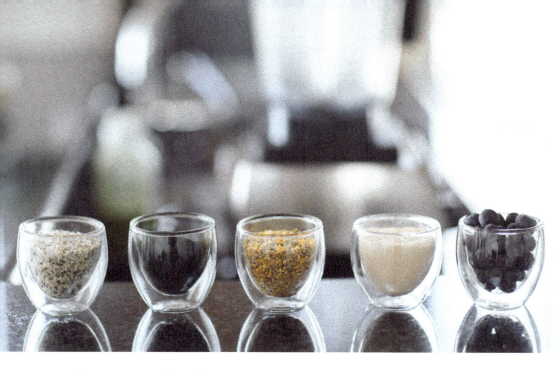

> *"Symptoms and conditions are communications from your body, telling you what it needs. That's what determines the best foods for you. A particular food belief system never trumps that—you can't impose a food belief system over your body's needs."*
>
> — Anthony Williams, *Medical Medium Life-Changing Foods*

## Sort Out Your Food Issues (and A Word on Detoxing)

When I was in high school, Mama Ruth and I embarked on our first official cleanse. If I remember correctly, it involved a lot of vegetable broth (we were vegetarians in those days), a lemon/water/cayenne concoction, and various juices. It lasted 14 long days and ended (for me, anyway) with a chocolate-chip cookie binge, which I promptly purged. While I was no stranger to long periods of time without food, the concept of cleansing to renew and heal my body or to discover which foods made me look and feel my best was lost on me at the time. I was in it for the quick weight loss and sense of control over my body, and my life, that restricting food provided for me.

I'm grateful that my healing journey has brought me to a place where I no longer need to restrict food to feel a sense of control over my body or my life. In the years since that first (fairly radical) cleanse, I've successfully completed numerous cleanses and I regularly practice food elimination as a way to stay in touch with my ever-evolving nutritional needs. Healing my relationship with food and making the choice to nurture, rather than punish, my body is a change that came through subtle shifts in both my thoughts and actions. It was a change in perspective, deeply connected to my highest intention of creating vibrant health in my body and happiness in my life. To honor that intention, I find it helpful to check in with myself before moving forward with significant changes to my daily diet. I do that by making sure the change I'm making is truly aligned with my intention of creating vibrant health. If I suspect it isn't, I turn my attention toward healing the part of myself seeking comfort in old, outmoded habits that don't support me. If the process of setting intentions is new for you and you're curious about how it works, check out my "Intention Starters" in the following chapter. Otherwise, I invite you to explore your own intentions for sorting out your food issues as you embark on the elimination diet.

While the structure I set out for you below is not a formal cleanse, when you make the choice to remove common toxic triggers from your diet, it frees your body up to do a more thorough job of removing impurities from your system, which can lead to both physical and emotional symptoms. Once we are no longer hiding behind our brain fog, bodily discomfort, and food addictions, the truth of our lives can emerge, and sometimes that can be a scary thing. We often have very good reasons for numbing ourselves to the difficult aspects of our lives, and when we strip that comfort away, we make space for our unresolved emotions to come up. This is a good time to go ahead and be gentle with yourself and reach out for support when you need it.

# How It Works

An elimination diet removes all the inflammatory and processed foods from your diet and allows you to get clear on what foods are toxic triggers for you. When we understand what foods are toxic triggers for us and take steps to alleviate or reduce them, energy levels increase, our minds get clearer, our sleep is deeper, and skin takes on a "lit from within" glow. If your own curiosity has led you to sorting out your food issues, I want to congratulate you on being willing to do the (sometimes hard) work of learning to listen to your body.

So, it's pretty simple: no gluten, dairy, eggs, soy, processed sugar, coffee, or alcohol for 23 days. Why 23 days? Antibodies, which are the proteins that your immune system makes when it reacts to foods, take about 21 to 23 days to turn over, so if you're sensitive to something 23 days is going to give you the full benefit of eliminating it from your diet. That said, I've had success with health coaching clients who followed a 10-day elimination diet, so if that sounds a bit more doable to you, feel free to start there. Either way, the next step is key. Following your elimination diet, you will move into the reintroduction phase. This reintroduction is key because it gives you the opportunity to discover exactly which foods trigger a response for you. If you were to add back every potential trigger food on day 24 and felt like something wasn't working well in your body, it would be *really* difficult to discover exactly which food it was!

Here's a quick snapshot of the foods you'll either be enjoying or holding off on while you sort out your food issues:

## Enjoy These Foods

- Greens and fresh vegetables (with a few exceptions)
- Whole fruits, fresh or frozen (with a few exceptions)
- Animal Protein: wild game (rabbit, pheasant, bison, venison, elk), lamb, duck, organic chicken and turkey, grass-fed beef

- Vegetable Protein: split peas, lentils, bee pollen, spirulina, blue green algae
- Fish: fresh or water-packed cold-water fish (trout, salmon, halibut, tuna, mackerel, sardines)
- Nuts & Seeds: hemp, sesame, and sunflower seeds; pecans, almonds, walnuts, cashews, pistachios, macadamia and Brazil nuts; lentils, quinoa
- Non-Gluten Grains & Starch: brown rice, millet, quinoa, amaranth, buckwheat
- Fermented foods (kimchi, sauerkraut)
- Unsweetened hemp and nut milks (almond, hazelnut, walnut, coconut)
- Fats and Oils: avocado, extra-virgin olive, flax, safflower, sesame, almond, sunflower, walnut, pumpkin, and coconut oils
- Sweeteners: raw honey, pure maple syrup, stevia, lucuma
- Drinks: filtered water, mineral water, green, white, and herbal teas, yerba mate

## Hold Off on These Foods

- Vegetables: corn, tomatoes, potatoes, eggplants, peppers
- Fruits: oranges, grapefruit, strawberries, grapes, bananas
- Animal Protein: eggs, raw fish, pork, sausage, cold cuts, canned meats, hot dogs, shellfish
- Vegetable Protein: soybean products (soy sauce, soybean oil, tempeh, tofu, soy milk, soy yogurt)
- Nuts & Seeds: peanuts, peanut butter, pistachios, macadamia nuts
- Dairy: milk, cheese, yogurt, butter, and non dairy creamers
- Sweeteners: refined sugar, white or brown sugar, high-fructose corn syrup, evaporated cane juice, agave
- Drinks: alcohol, coffee, soda

# It's Been 23 Days: You Feel Awesome—Now What?

This is the best part! You are in the reintroduction phase and you have the unique opportunity to find out exactly which foods disturb your body. The key is to test each food individually and to pay attention to not just the obvious signs of discomfort, such as a stomachache, but to more subtle signs like brain fog or an energy slump. You want to reintroduce one type of food from the "hold off" list into your daily meals each day. If you are choosing to reintroduce a gluten grain the first day, try having toast at breakfast or a sandwich at lunch. If you prefer to start with dairy, have some yogurt or cheese. Next, you will want to observe what happens over the next twenty-four hours. It can be very helpful to use a food diary for this phase as you notice the following:

- How do you feel immediately after eating it? Are there any sensations in your belly?
- Does anything happen shortly after you eat it, such as a runny nose or mucus in the throat (typical of milk), or fatigue, bloating, or headache (typical of gluten)?
- How are your energy levels?
- How is your poop the next day?
- How did you sleep? Was it a deep sleep or were you disturbed?
- How does your skin look? Any eruptions?
- How are your emotions the following day?

Any noticeable change in your physical or mental experience is an indication that you might be sensitive to that food. If you suspect this to be the case, eat that same food the next day and see if it provokes a reaction again. Just like the first day of reintroduction, notice what happens for a full day after eating the food, but note that the second-day reaction is likely to be less severe than the first. Repeat this same process with every food you wish to test from the "hold off" list. If you have a severe allergy to one of these foods, it will be quite obvious to you, but subtler reactions should not be dismissed.

# Rotate & Rethink

If your reaction to any of the foods you test is mild but still noticeable (slight fatigue, constipation, mood swings), you don't necessarily have to eliminate it forever, but you will still benefit from reducing the frequency of exposure to it. Following a rotation diet is a simple way of reducing the consequences of mild to moderate food sensitivities. This approach involves rotating your food choices so that you don't eat the irritating ones more than once every four days or so. That's a pretty easy tradeoff for feeling better overall.

> *"What you cultivate on the inside will begin to reverberate to your outside and will then be reflected back onto you through life's charm—the charm that comes from a life lived by someone who is thriving at the very core."*
> — Amanda Chantal Bacon, creator of Moon Juice

The concept of bio-individuality teaches us that there is no perfect way of eating that works for everyone. It also teaches us that what works for you today may not work for you tomorrow. There are a lot of dietary theories out there and it can be hard to figure out where to start. Lucky for you, there actually *is* a concept that truly works for anybody who tries it. Your path to vibrant health and radiant beauty doesn't come with a list of foods to avoid, but it does come with a list of foods to add in. This idea is based on a concept we learned in nutrition school called "crowding out," and it refers to the natural process that happens when you *add* more of the good stuff in first (think real food). Rather than focusing on what you *can't* have, you change the focus to abundance and curiosity as you expand your shopping list to include more of the nutrient-rich foods that help your body thrive. You'll notice over time that your cravings become redirected, making it easier to find your balance.

# Foods Your Body Wants You to Know About (This Is Your Shopping List)

By the time David "Avocado" Wolfe was a guest teacher at my nutrition school, my dog-eared copy of his book *Superfoods: The Food and Medicine of the Future* had become a trusted guidebook on my healing journey. The opportunity to study with the man who (literally) wrote the book on superfoods was pretty exciting to say the least. I like how he describes superfoods as a class of the most potent, super-concentrated, and nutrient-rich foods on the planet with the ability to tremendously increase the vital life force and energy of your body (he had me at "vital life force"). In this chapter I'm going to introduce you to some of the foods (and a sprinkling of adaptogens) that I consider super. I'm also going to share how easily I incorporate them into my daily life to support my own vibrant health and radiant beauty.

While you will recognize some of the foods that made my super list from your own pantry, you may not have been aware that these traditional foods hold such healing power. You may also run across a few things that blur the line between food and medicine that may not have made their way into your kitchen yet, but that's about to change. Along with an abundance of organic whole foods (the kind that grow in the ground), consider adding these foods to your shopping list (go all in or set your own pace). Not sure how to use them or where to buy them? No worries, I've got you covered. Check my "Stock Up" tips for the best ways to get these superfoods into your pantry *and* your body!

### Acai Berry = Glow Getting + Free Radical Fighting + Regenerating

Native to Central and South America, the purple acai berry gets its distinct color from high concentrations of the pigmented nutrients they contain, including impressive amounts of antioxidants. Antioxidants are free radical fighters, which means they help slow the process of free radical damage (or oxidative stress) that contributes to the wear and tear we attribute to aging. The external markers of oxidative stress (think dark spots, wrinkles, and sagginess) are all tied to free radical damage. Free radical damage not only makes us look older, it makes us feel older too (think achy joints, muscular pain, and brain fog). Consuming plenty of antioxidants is an ideal step on your path to vibrant health and radiant beauty.

**Stock Up:** While acai bowls at your local juice shop may be on trend, they can also be a sugar bomb, so proceed with caution. I find the easiest and most versatile way to include acai in my diet is to consume it in powder form and blend it into a (low sugar) juice or smoothie. Thrive Market (thrivemarket.com) is a wellness warrior's shopping dream come true. You can find most anything on their website at really good prices, including acai powder. You can also find it at your local health food store.

**Adaptogens = A Wellness Warrior's Secret Weapon**

Used in traditional Chinese and Ayurvedic medicine for centuries to boost energy and resilience, adaptogens support the health of our adrenal system by strengthening the body's response to stress. The most brilliant thing about adaptogens is that they "adapt" their function according to your body's specific needs. According to Dr. Frank Lipman, adaptogens enable the body's cells to access more energy, help cells eliminate toxic byproducts of the metabolic process, and help the body utilize oxygen more efficiently. One of my favorite ways to get to know the unique properties of adaptogens is to begin by incorporating them into my food or beverages one at a time and see how they make me feel. After that initial introduction, I start getting mixy in my kitchen and combine them to my desired effect. Here are some of my favorites:

### Ashwaganda = Calming + Happy Making + Sleep Supporting
This mineral-rich root is traditionally used to support thyroid function, improve sleep, and alleviate depression.

**Chaga = Happy Making + Glow Getting + Immunity Boosting**

Wild chaga mushroom is traditionally used to support glowing skin (yes, please!), longevity, and well-being.

**Cordyceps = Brain Boosting + Energizing + Hormone Balancing**

Cordyceps mushroom is traditionally used to balance hormones, increase stamina and energy, and improve both lung and brain function.

**Maca = Energizing + Hormone Balancing + Libido Lifting**

A (tasty) Peruvian root, energizing maca is traditionally used to balance hormones and increase mental stamina. It's also known to lift your mood *and* get you in the mood!

**Pearl = Glow Getting + Joy Promoting + Mineralizing**

A centuries-old beauty secret, this adaptogen is full of essential trace minerals, amino acids, and enzymes (hello, glow!).

**Reishi = Brain Boosting + Immunity Boosting + Liver Loving**

Regarded by many as the strongest immunity-boosting herb in the world, the reishi mushroom is also known to nourish the heart, brain, and liver while energizing the spirit.

**Schisandra Berry = Brain Boosting + Libido Boosting + Liver Loving**

A medicinal berry utilized in Traditional Chinese Medicine (TCM) for thousands of years, schisandra is most well known for boosting liver function, promoting mental clarity, and boosting libido.

**Stock Up:** The company Moon Juice (moonjuice.com) is a fantastic resource for purchasing all manner of adaptogens or adaptogenic blends (I'm partial to their Beauty and Sex Dusts), as well as other pantry staples. You can also find many of these products online at Thrive Market or at your local health food store. I sprinkle adaptogens into my coffee or tea, blend them into fresh-pressed juice or smoothies, and even stir them into tasty treats.

## Apple Cider Vinegar = Alkalizing + Glow Getting + Gut Healing

Made from apple cider that has undergone fermentation to form health-promoting probiotics and enzymes, raw apple cider vinegar (ACV) has been used for generations as a home remedy for everything from indigestion to allergies and clearing acne. Only raw apple cider vinegar has the "mother of vinegar" that makes the vinegar so beneficial. Made up of living nutrients and healthy bacteria, you can actually see it settled at the bottom of the bottle like sediment, so look for this when you make your purchase.

**Stock Up:** You can find organic ACV (Bragg's is my favorite) online at Thrive Market or at your local health food store. A traditional "wellness water" can be made by combining a shot of ACV with 8 ounces spring water and ideally consumed first thing in the morning. I also include ACV in my salad dressings, which can be a nice starting point if the idea of the wellness water doesn't seem palatable (it's not for everyone).

## Bee Pollen = Free Radical Fighting + Inflammation Taming + Wrinkle Warrior

Bee pollen is essentially all of the mineral matter inside of flowers that honeybees gather and bring back to the hive on their wings and legs. While that image alone makes me happy, bee pollen is also considered one of the most complete superfoods found in nature. It contains almost all of the nutrients required by the human body to thrive and is recognized as a medicine by the German board of health. While it's traditionally used to support immunity, fertility, and skin health, athletes in the know use bee pollen for muscle growth, stamina, and recovery from exercise. If you're new to enjoying bee pollen, it's a good idea to start out with a small dosage since some people may occasionally experience gastrointestinal irritation (think disaster pants).

**Stock Up:** Going local is best for bee products, so ideally you would want to check your local farmers market or health food store. Remember to bee kind by purchasing only organic and wild bee products and steer clear if bee products are not for you. I add bee pollen to smoothies, sprinkle over grain-free cereal, or combine with nut butter to spread on toast. It's also perfect as a dusting over tasty treats or eaten straight off a spoon if you like the taste (I do).

### Cacao = Brain Boosting + Bliss Inducing + Free Radical Fighting

Don't tell the other superfoods, but raw cacao might be my favorite! Not only is it super tasty, but this antioxidant superstar is also known to boost your metabolism, increase your focus, nourish your nervous system, boost your mood, *and* get you in the mood. It's full of phenylethylamine (PEA), a neurotransmitter produced naturally when we fall in love, and the "bliss chemical" anandamine, which is known to create feelings of attraction, excitement, or euphoria (yes, please!).

**Stock Up:** I like to keep raw cacao nibs, paste, and powder in my pantry. You can find these online at Thrive Market or at your local health food store. I'm also a huge fan of made-for-me-to-enjoy-immediately raw cacao treats! Some of my favorites are David "Avocado" Wolfe's Sacred Chocolate (sacredchocolate.com), the "Raw Remedies" line from Chocolatl (chocolatl.com), and the Raw Chocolate Lovers Bar from Medicinal Foods (medicinal-foods.com). Raw cacao has a special affinity for other superfoods and mixes well with medicinal mushrooms, gogi berries, maca, and more!

### Camu Camu = Glow Getting + Inflammation Taming + Happy Making

Grown on a shrub in the swamp or flooded areas of the Amazon rainforest, camu camu berries are one of the top vitamin C foods on the planet (hello, glow!). Fairly new to the global market, camu camu is traditionally used for eye and liver health, inflammation, mood, and more.

**Stock Up:** You can find camu camu powder online at Thrive Market or at your local health food store. The taste is quite sour, but powdered versions are easily tamed in smoothies or other beverages.

## Himalayan Pink Salt = Energizing + Hydration Helper + Mineralizing

Due to a lack of nutrient-rich soil, it's become harder for us to obtain the minerals and other trace elements that are essential to our health and well-being. Salt is a fantastic source, but unfortunately most of the table salt you find these days is stripped of its nutritional value and contains other potentially toxic ingredients such as anti-clumping and flowing agents, aluminum, and chlorine used for bleaching. Himalayan pink salt is mined from prehistoric seabeds and works as an electrolyte in your body, balancing fluid both inside and outside the cell walls. It regulates pH, stimulates digestive enzymes, and transports amino acids into the bloodstream.

**Stock Up:** You can find Himalayan pink salt at specialty food shops, online at Thrive Market, or at your local health food store. I use Himalayan pink salt in place of table salt in recipes or over vegetables. I also add a bit to fresh-pressed juices and wellness waters.

## Chia Seeds = Glow Getting + Energizing + Digestion Helper

A staple in ancient Aztec and Mayan diets, legend has it that warriors would fill up on energizing chia seeds before heading off to battle (wellness warriors, take note!). A rich source of plant-based omega-3 fatty acids, antioxidants, fiber, and minerals, chia seeds are pretty much perfect.

**Stock Up:** You can find organic chia seeds online at Thrive Market or at your local health food store. I love to use chia seeds in baking (great for paleo muffins) and for creating healthy desserts. They also blend well in a smoothie, but you'll want to consume it straight away before the seeds expand and make themselves into a pudding (also delicious).

### Coconut Oil = Gut Healing + Immunity Boosting + Metabolism Helper

An amazing source of healthy medium-chain fatty acids (MCFAs), coconut oil is high on my list of foods for taking an inside-out *and* outside-in approach to beauty (more on that later). Coconuts are rich in antimicrobial and antifungal properties, improve digestion and absorption of fat-soluble vitamins and amino acids, regulate and support healthy hormone production, and boost metabolism.

**Stock Up:** Refined or processed coconut oil can be bleached or chemically processed to improve its shelf life, so look for organic virgin coconut oil. You can find coconut oil online at Thrive Market or at your local health food store. I use coconut oil for cooking, baking, blending, and sometimes I eat it straight off a spoon because it's just that good.

### Collagen Protein = Beauty Boosting + Gut Healing + Joint Helper

Collagen supports the matrix of your bones, the lining of your arteries, heals cartilage, and supports tissue repair, promoting flexible joints and smooth, supple skin. The most traditional way to get collagen into your daily diet is making bone broth by boiling bones from grass-fed animals the way your grandmother used to do. If making your own bone broth isn't your thing, a terrific alternative is collagen powder from grass-fed cows.

**Stock Up:** I like the Bulletproof (bulletproof.com) brand of collagen protein because it's tasteless, making it ideal to add into your diet in a variety of ways. You can also find collagen protein online at Thrive Market or at your local health food store. I use collagen protein in my Bulletproof coffee and green tea lattes. It also blends well in a smoothie or many desserts.

### Chlorophyll = Digestion Helper + Liver Lover + Glow Getter

As you may recall from science class, chlorophyll is a type of plant pigment responsible for the absorption of light in the process of photosynthesis, which creates energy. Studies have shown that chlorophyll can bind to potential carcinogens and interfere with their absorption, which stops them from being circulated throughout the body (take that, toxins!). Chlorophyll promotes liver health, protects skin, speeds wound healing, and is a natural internal deodorizer.

**Stock Up:** I like to keep both unflavored and mint-flavored liquid chlorophyll on hand, both of which can be found online at Thrive Market or your local health food store. If you like the taste (it's earthy), it's easy to add unflavored chlorophyll to a glass of water. If you find that's not for you, try the mint-flavored version or make a (delicious) green lemonade by adding a tablespoon of chlorophyll, the juice of ½ a lemon (give or take), and a few drops of stevia to a 16-ounce glass of water.

## Fermented Food = Beauty Boosting + Gut Healing + Immunity Helper

Rich in lactobacilli and enzymes, alkaline forming, and loaded with vitamins, fermented foods like sauerkraut, kimchi, kombucha, and pickled veggies are ideal for creating vibrant health and radiant beauty. By eating fermented foods, you help to reestablish your inner ecosystem for healthy digestion and maintain your own enzyme reserve. This helps to eliminate toxins, rejuvenate your cells, and strengthen your immune system.

**Stock Up:** Look for raw fermented foods at your local farmers market or health food store, but don't be tricked by the sauerkraut in the deli section or by unrefrigerated pickles in the grocery aisle. Fermented foods need to be stored cold in order for the organisms to thrive. I try to eat at least one serving of fermented foods daily.

## Gogi Berries = Digestion Helper + Energizing + Mood Boosting

Legend has it that thousands of years ago monks in the Himalayan Mountains ate gogi berries steeped in hot water to aid meditation (I've tried it, it works!). Meditation benefits aside, gogi berries are traditionally used to fight depression, anxiety, and other mood disorders. They are also known for their ability to support digestion, energy production, and soothe stress.

**Stock Up:** Usually eaten dried or in powder form, I like to keep both on hand. You can find them online at Thrive Market or at your local health food store. I eat dried gogi berries by the handful, while the powdered form blends well into smoothies.

## Hemp Seed: Brain Boosting + Glow Getting + Poop Whisperer

This mineral rich, antioxidant superstar is one of my favorite ways to take an outside-in and inside-out approach to beauty. I love it not only because it's a potent source of plant protein and omega-3 fatty acids, but you can mix it with honey for a DIY gentle exfoliator. High in insoluble and soluble fiber, hemp seeds also help you poop.

**Stock Up:** You will find organic hemp seeds (sometimes called hemp hearts) online at Thrive Market or at your local health food store. I use hempseeds to make milk, blend into smoothies, and they are also delicious as a dusting for raw cacao treats.

## MCT Oil = Brain Boosting + Energizing + Metabolism Helper

With the popularity of Dave Asprey's "Bulletproof" coffee—an unlikely (and delicious) pairing of coffee, grass-fed butter, and MCT oil—you may be wondering what all the hype is about. MCT oil (an abbreviation of medium-chain triglyceride) is derived from coconuts or palm kernels with benefits ranging from increased energy and metabolism to better gut health and cognitive function. While coconut oil has MCTs in it, concentrated MCT oil is almost entirely MCTs and is considered the gold standard by devotees of the Bulletproof Diet. I like to keep both on hand.

**Stock Up:** Make sure you purchase high-quality MCT oil that clearly states what the ingredients are and how it was produced. While MCT oil can be derived from palm kernel oil, the production is connected to the destruction of orangutan habitats in Southeast Asia (let's not support that). Some MCT oils are also produced using solvents like hexane, which can leave residues (let's not support that either). My favorite trusted source is the Bulletproof brand "Brain

Octane Oil" available at bulletproof.com. You can also find MCT oil online at Thrive Market or at your local health food store. I use MCT oil in Bulletproof coffee, green tea lattes, and tasty treats.

## Wellness Teas = Alkalizing + Health Promoting

Growing up, Mama Ruth lined her pantry with all manner of loose-leaf teas stored in Mason jars. She always had just the right tea, no matter the occasion. While some of them were decidedly medicinal for my young palate, they were always steeped with the heartfelt intention to keep her girl well. Mama Ruth made the simple act of drinking tea a magical occasion, and a cup of tea continues to feel like magic in my life. You will *always* find these in my pantry:

### Burdock Root = Blood Purifier + Glow Getter + Lymph Lover

You might know burdock best as those small hooking burrs that stick themselves to your socks on a summer hike (pesky buggers). Those burrs come from the burdock plant, whose roots have been considered medicine for thousands of years. Traditionally used as a blood purifier, the active ingredients in burdock have been found to detoxify heavy metals, induce lymphatic drainage and detoxification, and promote blood circulation to help you get your glow on!

### Chamomile = Immunity Boosting + Stress Soothing + Sleep Whisperer

Chamomile is probably best known for its ability to soothe the mind and relax the body, but this antioxidant-rich brew boasts a variety of other health benefits. The phenolic compounds found in chamomile tea can help your body fight bacterial infections, and because of its antispasmodic and anti-inflammatory nature, it's perfect for reducing uncomfortable symptoms of menstruation or irritable bowel syndrome (think bloating and cramping). Chamomile tea can also be used topically for skin and hair health. A tea-soaked cotton round can be used as a toner to lessen the appearance of blemishes, and a final rinse with chamomile assures a good hair day.

### Dandelion = Detoxifying + Glow Getting + Liver Loving

Dandelion's bitter taste stimulates digestion, supports your liver, and helps you get your glow on. This backyard superfood also makes a tasty coffee replacement (my favorite is Dandy Blend). Dandelion plays well with fennel, and I love the bittersweet combo I get when I mix the two.

### Fennel = Bloat Busting + Detoxifying + Lung Loving

Traditionally used as a digestive aid, fennel also works as a cleanser and diuretic, keeping your kidneys and liver happy. It's often recommended for respiratory issues because it works as an expectorant, eliminating phlegm and mucus. I happen to love the licorice-like taste of fennel and find it particularly delicious as a palate cleanser.

### Hibiscus = Free Radical Fighting + Happiness Helper + Skin Firming

Traditionally used to relieve indigestion, constipation, and kidney ailments, skin-firming hibiscus also has a magical reputation as nature's Botox. I love hibiscus tea on its own (warm or cold) for a tart flavor or with a few drops of stevia for a sweeter treat.

### Lavender = Calming + Digestion Helper + Mood Balancing

Loved by many for its soothing aroma, lavender can stimulate the release of neurotransmitters that offset stress hormones and is traditionally used to induce relaxation.

Lavender can be helpful for anxiety, insomnia, stress, and depression. Lavender plays well with chamomile and I love a cup just before bed.

### Matcha = Brain Boosting + Happiness Helper + Metabolism Boosting

Super rich in chlorophyll, alkalizing matcha is a grassy powder made from Japanese whole leaf tea. It provides a steady, mood-boosting energy that increases your metabolic rate, helping you burn fat.

### Rooibos = Beauty Boosting + Bone Building + Heart Loving

According to the South African Rooibos Counsel, rooibos is not a true tea, but an herb. It contains minerals and the flavonoids orientin and luteolin, which support the growth of healthy bones (healthy bones are beautiful bones!). It's also rich in alpha hydroxy acids and antioxidants that help you get your glow on. Rooibos tea is quite tasty, making it easy to enjoy warm or cold on a regular basis.

### Stinging Nettle = Blood Building + Glow Getting + Mineralizing

Stinging nettle is a wild food traditionally used to treat allergies, anemia, and reproductive health. Rich in the beauty mineral silica, it's also a glow-getter. As its name suggests, this healing herbal tonic can make itself known with a painful sting! Mama Ruth grows it in her garden and has mastered the art of stingless cooking with it. I'm not quite as adventurous, but I do enjoy brewing up a pot of nettle tea, particularly in the spring when my allergies make themselves known.

**Smooth Move = Stimulating + Poop Whisperer**

Everybody loves to poop, so I keep this senna-based tea from Traditional Medicinals on hand for when I need a little extra support. Senna is a powerful but gentle leaf with laxative properties meant for occasional use to promote regularity. I find it particularly helpful to keep things moving during a cleanse or while traveling.

**Stock Up:** I'm a huge fan of Traditional Medicinals (traditionalmedicinals.com), not only for their selection of single and already-blended-for-you teas (it's like having Mama Ruth in your pantry!), but their Plant Power Journal is an amazing educational resource. You can also find organic tea online at Thrive Market or at your local health food store. A word of caution: wellness teas should be thought of as medicine, and while they are considered generally safe for overall health, it's important to check the packaging for any contraindications.

**Spirulina = Energizing + Free Radical Fighter + Muscle Repairing**

Consumed as a medicinal food dating back to the Aztec civilization of the 14th century, spirulina is a single-celled blue-green algae (think pond scum) that is cultivated around the world. It gained popularity in the mid-1970s when the World Food Conference declared it one of the "best foods for the future" to help fight malnutrition in areas of the world where food was scarce, and it became a staple for NASA's astronauts in space because of its superior nutritional profile. Arguably one of the most nutrient-dense foods on the planet, I've enjoyed spirulina since Mama Ruth started blending it into our smoothies decades ago. With a full spectrum of amino acids, it's considered a complete protein and rich source of vital nutrients. If you find you don't love the taste, most blended green powders on the market contain spirulina and you can start there.

**Stock Up:** Not all spirulina products are created equal, and because this superfood is known to absorb heavy metals and toxins from its environment, it's super important to make sure yours is from a clean source. According to Dr. Axe, these brands are among the best in terms of organic farming and testing for toxic metals: Nutrex, Organic Burst, Triquetra Health, and Spiru-Blue. You can find spirulina online at Thrive Market, Amazon, or Moon Juice, as well as at your local health food store. I blend spirulina into my smoothies and use them as a dusting for tasty treats.

## Sprouts = Alkalizing + Free Radical Fighting + Nutrient Enhancing

It probably goes without saying, but Mama Ruth considered sprouts a staple in our home and remains an avid sprout farmer to this day (I am too). Proponents of raw and "living" foods believe that sprouts, which are *truly* alive at the time of consumption, impart their life energy and vitality to our systems when we eat them. Sprouting is the process of germinating seeds to create a living, growing food source with an abundant supply of enzymes and vital nutrients. Sprouting is also the perfect upgrade to foods you may already be eating like nuts, seeds, or grains. These foods contain inherent toxic inhibitors that protect the plant from germination until the ideal conditions are present, and while this natural protective phenomenon ensures the plant's survival, it can wreak havoc in our digestive systems. When you soak nuts, seeds, and grains, the germination process begins, allowing the enzyme inhibitors to be deactivated and increasing available nutrition. A study by the Johns Hopkins School of Medicine shows that three-day-old broccoli sprouts contain 10 to 100 times the cancer-fighting compounds found in mature broccoli.

**Stock Up:** I purchase all my certified organic, non-GMO seeds from the company Sprout House (sprouthouse.com), as well as all my sprouting supplies. If you are purchasing sprouts, try your local farmers market or health food store and have fun trying a wide variety of sprouted seeds. My favorites are sunflower, radish, and broccoli, but I truly love them all! You can also find already sprouted (or "activated") nuts and seeds online at Thrive Market or your local health food store.

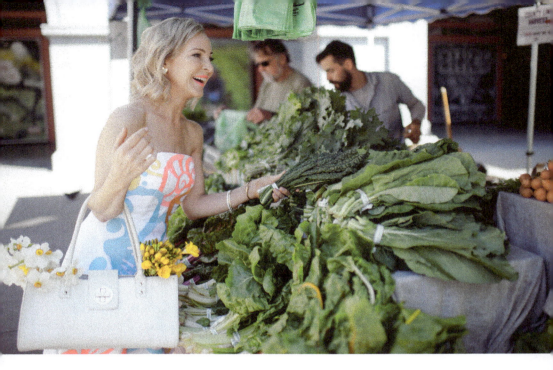

Every moment of every day our cells are breathing, working, and generating waste. The air we breathe, the water we drink, the food we eat, the products we use in our homes and on our bodies are all loaded with toxic chemicals. Some of us even have mercury leaking from our very own mouths. Taking steps to upgrade your lifestyle will give you an immediate boost in vitality and will support you on your path to vibrant health and radiant beauty!

**Your Upgraded Lifestyle in Action**

- Commit to eating an organic, whole-foods diet whenever possible (avoiding commercially raised meat is a nonnegotiable!).
- Filter your water.
- Reduce toxins in your everyday routine.
- Consider having any dental amalgams (safely) removed by a biologic dentist. Not sure? Open wide and look for metal. Having your amalgams removed will reduce your exposure to heavy metals.

Notice in your home and work environments where you are exposed to unnecessary toxins and take steps to reduce them. A great place to start is by swapping out your household cleaning supplies and personal care products. You can find a lot of great information available online about making your home and life toxin-free. Here are a few basic recipes and techniques to get you started!

**All-Purpose Cleaner**

- 2 cups white distilled vinegar
- 2 cups water
- Essential oil (optional)

You can use this all-purpose cleaner on hard surfaces such as countertops and kitchen floors.

**Glass Cleaner**

- ¼ cup vinegar
- 1 quart water

Mix together in spray bottle. Spray on glass and wipe with lint-free cloth.

**Soft Scrub**

- 2 cups baking soda
- ½ cup to ⅔ cup liquid castile soap
- 4 teaspoons vegetable glycerin
- 5 drops antibacterial essential oil (optional)

Mix together and store in a sealed glass jar. Use this on kitchen counters, stoves, bathtubs, and sinks.

**Furniture Polish**

- ¼ cup olive oil
- ¼ cup distilled vinegar
- 20 drops lemon essential oil

Shake well and dip a clean, dry cloth into the polish and rub wood in the direction of the grain.

Use a soft brush to work the polish into corners or tight places.

## Clean Beauty - Where to Start?

Our skin absorbs what we put on it, so we need to be super diligent about what we stock our medicine cabinets, shower shelves, and makeup bags with. The beauty industry is essentially unregulated, and this means that cosmetic companies can legally put all manner of toxic ingredients (even known carcinogens!) into the products we use every day and they don't even have to list them on the label. Even if trace amounts of toxins were "safe," as the beauty industry would have us believe, it's easy to underestimate the amount and number of toxins that you are actually ingesting and absorbing from personal care products. Even if a chemical isn't so harmful that we feel its effects immediately, some bio-accumulate in the body, taking their toll over time. When you are dealing with chemicals that are carcinogenic, interfere with hormones (endocrine disruptors), or are toxic to your nervous system, the goal is to minimize exposure as much as possible. With so many harmful chemicals lurking out there, it can be a bit overwhelming. So, where to start? Look for alternatives to the ten most common and toxic chemicals likely hiding out in your skin care, makeup, or body products.

**Kick these to the curb:**

- **Parabens:** Pharmaceutical companies started using parabens to preserve products in the 1920s. Parabens are used to suppress microbial growth in everything from shampoo, conditioner, perfume, toothpaste, soaps, and other hygiene products. Parabens are estrogenic, meaning they compete with estrogen for binding sites in the body, potentially affecting hormonal balance. Be on the lookout for methylparaben, ethylparaben, propylparaben and butylparaben on the label, and avoid these products.

- **Sodium Lauryl Sulfates (SLS):** Your shampoo, body wash, and facial cleanser very likely contain SLS or its slightly gentler alternative, sodium laureth sulfate. The main problem with this ingredient is that it's corrosive and wears away at the protective lining of your skin. Another unpleasant effect of SLS is skin aging due to the protein-denaturing properties of this ingredient. Skin aging as a result of sun exposure is believed to occur because of protein denaturation.

- **Mineral Oil:** Mineral oil is a by-product of the production of crude oil. Our skin doesn't absorb mineral oil well and it can clog your pores, but it isn't just a cosmetic issue. Mineral oil is often tainted with other chemicals during the refining process, none of which you want to be using on your skin.

- **Phthalates:** Phthalates are a group of chemicals that are disruptive to the endocrine system, which can lead to developmental, reproductive, and neurological damage. Specifically, phthalates are shown to worsen a woman's egg quality and quantity. Phthalates are found in everything from deodorant to nail polish and scented lip balm.

- **Oxybenzone:** Most sunscreens contain a harmful chemical called oxybenzone, which some studies have shown to be carcinogenic and hormone-mimicking. Switching to a sunscreen with zinc oxide can give you protection from the sun without the worry. Look for one that also contains skin-healing ingredients like avocado oil and aloe vera.

- **Lead:** Lead is a proven neurotoxin linked to miscarriage and reduced fertility. It can show up in our foundation, lipsticks, and whitening toothpaste. It isn't actually added as an ingredient, but it makes its way into these products through contamination, commonly through color additives. The best way to avoid lead is to buy makeup from companies that make products in small batches and to buy products colored naturally with fruit pigments or alkanet root.

- **Aluminum:** Classified as a neurotoxin, aluminum is commonly used in antiperspirant deodorants and has been linked to breast cancer, Alzheimer's, and other brain disorders. There are a ton of natural deodorants out there (you've likely tried one that you didn't love), so do some experimenting and find one that works for you.

- **Triclosan:** Triclosan is commonly found in hand sanitizer and is included as an antibacterial agent. Bacteria are necessary for our health, and being in the habit of constantly removing bacteria from our bodies through the overuse of antibiotics and hand sanitizers is not health-promoting. For everyday purposes, good old soap and water does the trick.

- **PEG Compounds:** Polyethylene glycols (PEGs) are petroleum-based compounds and are a common ingredient in cosmetics used to thicken, soften, and gelatinize the product. The main issue with PEGs is that they are often contaminated with ethylene oxide and 1,4-dioxane. Ethylene oxide is a known human carcinogen that is potentially harmful to the nervous system and human development. 1,4-dioxane is a possible human carcinogen that can remain in the environment for long periods of time without degrading. PEG compounds enhance the penetration of other ingredients into your skin, which is great if the ingredients are healthy, but not so great if they aren't. The number next to PEG on a label indicates how many units of ethylene glycol they comprise. The lower the number, the more easily the product absorbs into your skin.

- **Hydroquinone:** This ingredient is commonly used in products that lighten skin, so if you are currently using something for age spots, sun damage, or acne scars, check the label for this ingredient. Studies on animals have produced evidence that hydroquinone could be carcinogenic when taken orally, and since this ingredient has the ability to penetrate deep into the skin, topical use is concerning as well. Using hydroquinone long term can also decrease your skin elasticity—and nobody wants that! There are several natural ingredients that you can use to lighten and brighten your skin. Skip the hydroquinone and look for products containing licorice root, vitamin C, and turmeric.

Overwhelmed by the prospect of throwing out your entire makeup cabinet and starting over? Try replacing things as they run out, and if you are concerned about a particular brand, do a cross-reference on the Environmental Working Group's website, Skin Deep (www.ewg.org/skindeep). If the product is a level 1 or level 2, it's probably not worth throwing away immediately, but if it's a "code red" toss it straight away! Keep in mind that big beauty companies are now using a strategy called "greenwashing" and that even labels like "cruelty free" and "organic" are beginning to lose some of their meaning. This is why it's important to check the back of the package for a product's *actual* ingredients.

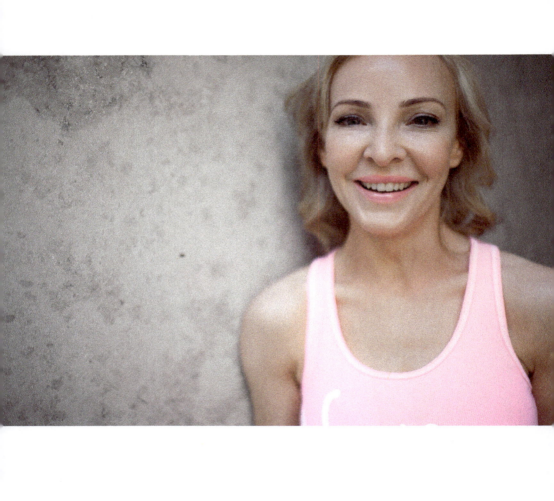

# Chapter Three
# Movement Is a Gift

*"Movement in your body creates movement in your life."*
— Erin Stutland,
author of *Mantras In Motion* and creator of *The Movement*

**I was about** eight years old when I was first inspired to exercise watching my Great-grandma Audi perform her nightly calisthenics. I perched myself on the back of the couch and observed her movements, fascinated by the rhythm. It was orderly and precise, something consistent that you could count on, and I craved that in my life. There were leg lifts, sit-ups, side bends, arm circles, and all manner of stretching. She never missed a day, which was pretty amazing for a polio survivor who had suffered greatly for the gift of walking on her own, without the rehabilitative brace she had worn in her younger years. I took her cue and started making up routines, performing them each night before bed like my own sacred ritual.

I wasn't one for organized sports—I was too shy for that kind of thing—but I sure did love finding new ways to move my body. It started with mimicking Grandma Audi's calisthenics and later, practicing yoga alongside my mom, as we listened to the instructions coming from her *Yoga for Health* record in our living room. Early on,

I wasn't so caught up in the idea of exercising to make my body look a certain way; it was about the pure joy of movement. In the '80s I adored Jane Fonda, leg warmers, and dance aerobics. If you are picturing me with feathered hair and a leotard, you are spot on. I even became fascinated, for a time, with women bodybuilders. I saved up my allowance to purchase a bench and free weights, and was super proud to ask my family members, "Want to feel my muscles?" I still do this. I discovered running in high school and could often be found challenging the hills in my rural hometown of Bodega, California. More and more I began to recognize, and crave, those euphoric moments that came to me when I laced up my sneakers and hit the pavement (hello, endorphins!).

My relationship with exercise has occasionally been a difficult one. Over the decades I struggled with an eating disorder, I often used over-exercising as a tool to distract myself. Countless hours sweating it out was a way for me to not be fully present in my body and in my life. Focusing on the perpetually just-out-of-reach goal of attaining my "ideal" body allowed me the freedom of not looking too closely at the things in my life that were crying out for attention. Who had time for all that life stuff when there was the urgent matter of decreasing the size of my thighs? If I distracted myself enough, those things could wait forever. Or so I hoped.

When I injured my cervical spine in 2008, escaping through movement was no longer an option for me. The escape I'd come to rely on was the very thing that led to my injury, setting the stage for chronic pain that I now manage daily. It was a struggle to release my outmoded patterns, but eventually I came to understand that in order to heal and feel at home in my body again (or maybe for the first time), I would need a new approach. Along with the physical therapy I was prescribed, I began exploring more "alternative" healing modalities including acupuncture, Emotional Freedom Technique (EFT), and energy medicine. I also rekindled my meditation practice and began seeing a psychotherapist. While nerve damage led to my decision to undergo surgery, the combination of practices I was using had a healing effect far beyond the original intent. I developed a more compassionate relationship with my body and learned that if I was willing to listen, my body held the answers to pretty much everything. Yours does too.

Movement is still a place for me to settle back into myself, to gain clarity, and move forward in my life, but balance can be tricky. Over time I've come to regard my habit of escaping through movement as a gift. It's a little reminder of how easy it can be to lose focus, to slip back into our comfort zones and live life on autopilot. Today, when I find myself focused on my body at the expense of other areas in my life, I recognize the need to slow down and breathe, to pay attention to whatever it is I'm having a hard time being present for. It's a reminder of my intention to feel, digest, and move through my experience of life. Cultivating a mindful movement practice has allowed me to honor movement as the gift that it is, while supporting my intention to remain present in my body and more able to hear its important messages.

You can use movement to strengthen and heal your body, to gain clarity, and to gather momentum to move forward in your life. As you become more self-confident through movement, you become motivated and empowered to address other obstacles in your life as well. Show up for your workouts ready to be moved—not just physically, but mentally and spiritually as well. Make movement a part of you. Move for the joy of it. Move because you *can* move.

So, what moves you?

## Creating Your Mindful Movement Practice

Jon Kabat Zinn, MD, founder of Mindfulness-Based Stress Reduction, defines mindfulness as "paying attention, on purpose, in the present moment, and nonjudgmentally." A mindful movement practice is taking these same principles and applying them to the way you move your body. When we think of mindful movement, often the more "Zen" practices come to mind (think yoga, Pilates, or Qigong), but slowing down and focusing attention can help improve the action and outcome of whatever workout you choose to do.

The idea is to be fully aware of your flow of energy, movement, and presence. The practice of mindfulness will increase your kinesthetic awareness, your ability to coordinate motion, and your awareness of where your body is in relation to time and space. This awareness allows you to gauge proper form and technique, giving you a better sense of where you might be compensating or imbalanced in your movement patterns. This awareness can reduce your risk of injury by allowing you to feel the sensations of pain or discomfort and properly assess their meaning.

There's another bonus to approaching your workouts with mindfulness (I think you'll like this one): better results! According to Dr. Kristin Race, PhD, an expert on brain-based mindfulness solutions, "mindfulness helps train the prefrontal cortex, the part of the brain that creates a calm and alert state of mind … and perform at our best." You also activate the insular cortex of the brain, which improves the communication between the body and the mind. When you focus on your muscle working, you actually increase the degree to which it contracts, and a larger part of your brain responsible for that muscle is activated. Numerous clinical studies have shown that intentionally focusing attention on the muscles you're working leads to increased muscle contraction and better results. So, take that mindfulness of yours to a Booty Barre class, the weight room, or out for a run! Here's how:

**Feel Your Body:** Before beginning any exercise, pause and bring awareness to your physical body. Take a few deep in- and out-breaths. Feel your bones, muscles, organs, tissue, and skin. How does your body feel? Do you have any pain or discomfort? Is your energy low? If you are not physically or mentally prepared to exercise, wait until you are (this is where that "nonjudgmental" part kicks in). Feeling good? Mindfully move on to the next step.

**Feel Your Space:** Allow your awareness to expand out to your environment and fill up the space that you're going to be moving through. Ideally, your space should be distraction-free, leaving you solely focused on the activity at hand. The ideal doesn't always happen, so be mindful that the more outside distractions you encounter, the more you will need to focus your attention on the task at hand (it's good practice anyway).

**Set Your Intention:** Before beginning your exercise, pause briefly to set a clear intention for what you are about to do. We set intentions in yoga all the time, but it's not as common with other forms of fitness. Let's change that! Creating an intention focuses your mind on what you're doing, increasing your chances for success. Intentions can be clear and specific like stating "I am training for a 5k" before you head out for a run, or a simple word or phrase you'd like to align yourself with like "I am creating strength." Need help with this one? Go to "Intention Starters" below for tips.

**Mind Your Breath:** Your breath infuses your body with oxygen and prana (life force) and is the connection between your body, mind, and spirit. The more deeply you breathe, the deeper you allow this connection to become. This is key to creating your mindful movement practice! With each exercise, strive to maintain awareness of the inflow and outflow of your breath, anchoring yourself into the present moment. You can experiment to find a breathing cadence that aligns with the exercise you are doing. Regardless of its variations, continue to come back to the breath.

**Mind Your Posture:** A neutral spine position creates the optimal spinal alignment for any physical activity. Without a neutral spine, you throw off your body's natural flow of energy, increasing the likelihood of injury and decreasing the benefits of exercise. Not sure what a "neutral" spine position feels like? Try this: Stand with your feet hip-width apart, toes pointing forward. Allow your pelvis to be in a neutral position, so that your low back isn't overarched or super flat (be sure that your tailbone isn't tucked under). Roll your shoulders up, and then down and back. Your shoulders are away from your ears, and your chest is open. Lift the crown of your head up toward the ceiling, standing tall, in perfect alignment with your head over your hips, over your heels. You are now standing with a neutral spine.

## Intention Starters

An intention is a guiding principle for how you want to show up in the world. It's a journey toward a more positive version of yourself, reflected in your actions. If you're focusing your mind on a specific intention during a meditation, you are bringing it to your focused mind, your thoughts, your heart, and in turn, helping to bring it into reality. You can do the same thing with your movement practice. You'll want to set aside some time for the following exercise and grab yourself a pen and paper. Take a few deep in- and out-breaths to quiet your mind and tune in to yourself. When you're ready, ask yourself the following questions:

## The Questions

Q. What matters most to you?

Q. What would you like to build, create, or nurture in your life?

Q. What would you like to let go of?

Q. What word(s) would you like to align yourself with?

Q. What are you grateful for?

## The Answers (the "Why" to the "What")

I like to approach these questions intuitively, letting my answers be the first thing that comes to mind. Once I have my answer, I find it helpful to dig a little deeper by asking myself the "why" to my "what." This exercise generally goes one of two ways: my "why" makes me feel more strongly connected to my answer, or it makes me rethink my answer altogether (either way is good!). Give it a try and see what comes up for you.

A. What matters most to me is that I'm present for my life. Why? Being present for my life allows me to feel a deeper connection to myself and to those I love.

A. I would like to create vibrant health in my body. Why? Experiencing vibrant health in my body allows me the freedom to move forward in my life.

A. I would like to let go of negative self-talk about my body. Why? I understand that the stories we tell ourselves about our bodies or our lives shape our reality. I choose to shape a positive reality for myself.

A. The word(s) I would like to align myself with are balance and strength. Why? When my body is out of balance, my life feels out of balance. Creating balance and strength supports me in my life as a whole.

A. I am grateful for the gift of movement. Why? There was a time when I was unable to move my body without experiencing a debilitating amount of pain, and this experience allowed me to appreciate movement as the gift that it is.

## Putting It All Together: Create Your Intention

Q. What matters most to you? A. What matters most to me is that I'm present for my life. Why? Being present for my life allows me to feel a deeper connection to myself and to those I love. *My intention is to be present and focused, to show up for this workout.*

Q. What would you like to build, create, or nurture in your life? A. I would like to create vibrant health in my body. Why? Experiencing vibrant health in my body allows me the freedom to move forward in my life. *My intention for practicing yoga today is to create vibrant health in my body.*

Q. What would you like to let go of? A. I would like to let go of negative self-talk about my body. Why? I understand that the stories we tell ourselves about our bodies or our lives shape our reality. I choose to shape a positive reality for myself. *My intention is to love my body, without judgment, throughout today's movement practice.*

Q. What word(s) would you like to align yourself with? A. The words I would like to align myself with are balance and strength. Why? When my body is out of balance, my whole life feels out of balance. Creating balance and strength supports me in my life as a whole. *My intention for practicing Pilates today is to create balance and strength in my body, mind, and spirit.*

Q. What are you grateful for? I am grateful for the gift of movement. Why? There was a time when I was unable to move my body without experiencing a debilitating amount of pain, and this experience allowed me to appreciate movement as the gift that it is. *My intention during my movement practice today is to recognize that every opportunity to move my body is a gift.*

## Shift Your Mindset: Movement & Mantras

*"Pairing affirmations with movement sends a new message to every cell in your body; the words that you are saying become your actual beliefs and your beliefs influence the actions you are willing to take in your life."*

— Erin Stutland

I'm a huge fan of Erin Stutland, the inspiring creator of The Movement—a unique fitness program combining cardio/dance/yoga/kickboxing moves with life-affirming, say-it-out-loud mantras designed to create movement in your body, and in your life. I love how Erin describes her program as kind of "Jane Fonda meets Tony Robbins" (she had me at Jane Fonda). I was first introduced to Erin's work through her "Say it, Sweat it, Get it" challenge (it's free and it's awesome). Aside from it being a fantastic introduction to her programs, it was a reminder to me of how powerful setting intentions and saying positive affirmations, or mantras, can be. This reminder couldn't have come at a better time for me. Shortly before learning about Erin's program, I was diagnosed with something called spondy (short for spondylolisthesis)—a forward displacement of the vertebra in my lumbar spine. If it sounds like it hurts, it does. It also forced me to rethink the way I'd been moving my body. Again.

This new diagnosis felt like a huge setback for me. In the years since my cervical spine injury, I'd slowly regained the strength I'd lost from nerve damage and muscle atrophy. While I did have the occasional flare-up since undergoing surgery and had made the choice to put away my running shoes, I was grateful to be in a place where I felt a certain amount of freedom in my movement. I was devoted to Tracy Anderson's Method, had returned to my beloved yoga practice, and had just discovered Booty Barre, taught by the motivating team at Maiden Lane Studios in San Francisco. I was feeling strong and fit, maybe even a little sexy (a known side effect of Booty Barre), but had to admit to some chronic low back pain that wasn't resolving. I knew from my previous experience that it's best to get to the bottom of any lingering pain sooner rather than later, and I'm glad I did. Sometimes we put nagging symptoms on the back burner, but if you catch imbalance in your body early on, you have a way better chance of course correcting and having a quicker healing outcome.

Remember what you learned about food and bio-individuality in the first chapter? This is what bio-individuality in movement looks like. In my case, having spondy meant that my spine wasn't super stable, and some of the movements I was performing regularly were no longer appropriate for me. As much as I loved my current routine, it was time for me to find a way to move my body that accommodated my changing needs. I wasn't exactly sure where to start, but having a dog in your life makes getting out for a walk on the daily a must, so that's what I did. This is where Erin's philosophy of combining movement and mantras stepped in and pretty much changed everything for me.

As part of her "Say it. Sweat it. Get it." challenge, Erin created a little something called the Soul Stroll—an upbeat playlist with her favorite mantras layered in. I laced up my walking shoes, put my ear buds in, and hit *play*.

"I am strong now. I have all that I need."

It just so happened that the words to this particular Soul Stroll really resonated with me. Okay, not so much at first. The truth was that I didn't believe that I was strong. In fact, I was mostly scared and in a good amount of pain. But, I went with the "fake it until you make it" strategy and said the words. Whispered really, "I am strong now." My body didn't feel strong, but I said it anyway. Then I realized that even though my body wasn't particularly strong in this moment, I actually am strong. I'd faced some pretty difficult challenges in my life and proven to myself time and time again that I *am* strong. I repeated the mantra louder than a whisper: "I am strong now." I emphasized the word "now" and something changed for me; I began to feel that right here, right now in the present moment, I was strong.

I continued to follow Erin's lead and repeated the words she spoke in my ear: "I have all that I need." Again, I didn't fully believe that I had all that I needed, but I said the words. I said them out loud again and again: "I am strong now. I have all that I need." I began to feel that I actually did have all that I needed. I had access to knowledgeable professionals who could help me navigate this whole spondy thing. I wasn't alone in my struggle, so why did I initially feel like I was? Because sometimes when we feel fear, we get stuck in our stories about who we are and what we have available to us. When something gets challenging, we have a tendency to want to run from it. We run into our stories to get out of this discomfort. Even if our stories are no longer true, even if our stories were never true, they are our stories and there can be a certain amount of comfort in that. The mantras don't allow you to do that, they keep you anchored into the present moment, where anything can be true for you. Did I feel a little silly walking my dog, saying mantras out loud for the Universe to hear? Of course I did, but mantras are catchy little things that create an empowering dialogue between your body, mind, and spirit. By the end of my first Soul Stroll, I was practically shouting them!

So, how does this mantra thing work? There is a long history of scholarly disagreement on the meaning of mantras. The Sanskrit word "mantra" consists of the root *man–*, "to think," and the suffix *–tra*, "designing tools or instruments." A literal translation would be "instrument of thought." Many believe that when spoken or chanted, mantras direct the healing power of prana (life-force energy), and in traditional Vedic practices are used to energize and access spiritual states of consciousness. The tapping of the tongue on the roof of the mouth sends messages and vibrations to your brain, and then the whole body, to effect very real change. I like to think of a mantra as a seed for energizing an intention. Mantras like "I am strong" or "I let go of the old" can help you maintain a connection to the state you wish to cultivate during your mindful movement practice. However you choose to think of a mantra, the result is that they leave you feeling strong, capable, focused, and motivated. Sounds pretty good, right?

## Create Your Mantra

> *"It's my time*
> *My vision is clear*
> *I can feel my power*
> *Right now right here ... "*
> — Erin Stutland

Your mantra is an authentic, individualized expression of a desire you wish to bring into your personal experience. Aligning your mantra with the intention you've set for your movement practice is a powerful way to create transformation in any area of your life that you choose.

Step 1: Get clear on your focus.

Step 2: Imagine that the change you seek is already part of your reality.

Step 3: Turn what you've imagined into a declarative statement.

**Focus:** You can narrow down an area of your life you'd like to focus on (health, relationships, finances, etc.) by either jumping ahead to chapter seven and working with the Circle of Life exercise or setting aside some quiet time to journal—whatever works for *you*!

**Feel It:** The next step is to imagine that you already have what you are looking to attract as part of your reality. For example, if the area I wanted to focus on was my health and my intention was to practice yoga to create vibrant health in my body, I would imagine myself experiencing vibrant health. I would connect with this feeling, noticing all the subtle details, until I could actually feel deep in my cells that I was experiencing vibrant health.

**You've Got This:** The final step is to turn what you've imagined into a declarative statement. If I were to use my intention of creating vibrant health, my declarative statement might be "I am creating vibrant health." Focus, feel it, declare it … ta da! You've got your mantra. Need a little help getting your mantra juices flowing? I consider Erin Stutland, Danielle LaPorte, Kris Carr, and Gabby Bernstein to be my own personal Superheroes of inspiration. When in doubt, I turn to them:

> *"I stay in the flow."*
> — Erin Stutland

> *"I feel into the bliss of my core. I increase my capacity for more."*
> — Danielle LaPorte, *The Desire Map*

> *"I love to breathe. Oxygen is sexy."*
> — Kris Carr, best-selling author, wellness activist and cancer survivor

> *"Your presence is your power."*
> — Gabby Bernstein, *Miracles Now*

# Your Mantra in Action

*"Pumping pedals, pumping pedals."*
— Mama Ruth, 1977

So you nailed your mantra down—now what? During my yoga practice, I often chant the words "*Sa, Ta, Na, Ma*" (birth, life, death, rebirth). I love the simple reminder of the circle of life and its ability to bring me to a place of inner calm. I also like to use the mantra "your presence is your power" during Pilates, because it feels right for the flow of movement. I don't necessarily repeat my mantra the entire time I'm practicing. I find a cadence that works with my breath and movement, pause for a time, then return to the words when I'm ready (you'll get the hang of it). What feels perfect for one workout might not feel perfect for another, so you'll definitely want to play with this.

The other day I was on the recumbent bike doing a 20-minute HIIT routine (that stands for high-intensity interval training and as the name suggests, it's intense). Instead of setting an intention and practicing a mantra, I put my headphones on and pedaled to some hip-hop. Over the course of this 20-minute workout, I pedal at a moderate speed for 90 seconds and then crank up the intensity, pedaling as hard and fast as I can for 30 seconds, before returning back to a moderate speed. I repeat this cycle for 20 minutes and the 30-second intervals start to get really, really hard. I was listening to my music, pushing through those 30 seconds when I noticed I was repeating the words "pumping pedals, pumping pedals" in my head. I laughed at the memory of my very first mantra and then I killed those 30 seconds! I credit my Mama Ruth and her resourcefulness as a single young mother saving up her quarters to keep us in clean clothes for this early lesson in mindfulness. A washer/dryer would have been a luxury for us in those days, and a car wasn't in the budget either. Back then we had bikes with baskets on the back and we had laundry—sometimes a lot of it. I'm not exactly sure how far the trip to the Laundromat actually was, but to my eight-year-old legs it was *far*. Halfway through the trip I'd inevitably start to slow my pace, maybe even whine a bit about the whole darn thing. That's when Mama Ruth would suggest we play our game and had us repeat out loud "pumping pedals, pumping pedals." It was silly, it was fun, and it worked. I wasn't paying attention to my too-tired legs. I wasn't on my way to the Laundromat for a dreaded chore. I was pumping pedals. That's all I was doing: pumping pedals. Sometimes you start a workout without a mantra and your mantra finds you anyway.

Back to the part where I told you that I don't *always* use mantras during my workouts. While I love the process of setting intentions (that's a nonnegotiable for me) and using mantras, I also love to break my own rules so that my life (and my workout) doesn't feel too rigid. I like to think of intentions and mantras as some of the tools in my toolbox, available to me any time I need them.

## Core Strength, Personal Transformation, and How to Not Pee Your Pants

Want to keep your lovely lady bits inside your body where they belong? Of course you do! Then you are going to want to pay attention to the health of your core muscles. Yes, really. It's called "pelvic organ prolapse" and unfortunately it's a thing. Prolapse is when one or more of the pelvic structures (think uterus, bladder, vagina, and/or rectum) fall or slip out of place. If this is the first time you are hearing about this, go ahead and let it sink in. Core dysfunction is a term used to describe "unwanted issues" caused by a weakening of your core muscles. While pelvic organ prolapse certainly makes the top of the "unwanted issues" list, I consider a leaky bladder and/or disaster pants (yes, I'm talking poop) pretty high on the list as well. All movement relies on the core and pelvic floor muscles to provide stability and control. If you live an active lifestyle where walking, squatting, jumping, pushing, pulling, and lunging are a normal part of your daily routine, you are naturally using these essential muscles all day long. If you aren't, it's probably time to start.

Are you at risk for "unwanted issues"? While giving birth is a common cause of core dysfunction, any repeated downward pressure on your pelvic organs, without support from your pelvic floor muscles, can put you at risk. What does downward pressure look like? If you put downward pressure on a toothpaste tube that isn't capped, the toothpaste would squirt out—except "toothpaste" isn't toothpaste, it's an organ. Yikes, right? If you've been associating core strength with the ability to rock your bikini, you're not alone. I have to admit I kind of thought that too. As it turns out, my own toned tummy was more a source of pride than helpful in my daily activities or preventing injury, and while I'm not admitting to *actually* peeing my pants, I've sure had some close calls. When I was experiencing a lot of lower-back pain prior to my spondy diagnosis, I started noticing that it became harder and harder to "hold it" when I really had to go. At the time, I didn't understand the connection, but I do now and I want you to understand it too!

Body mechanics, or the way you use your body to complete your daily physical activities, are super important to consider in both prevention and treatment of core dysfunction. This includes things like straining to lift something heavy (or to pass a difficult bowel movement); not balancing your daily run with a core-strengthening routine; lack of physical activity; and even standing or sitting with poor posture. Having embraced movement at a young age, it never occurred to me that I didn't have the whole body mechanics thing down. As it turned out, I'd actually spent decades moving my body in some pretty inefficient ways, many of which contributed to my chronic pain and left unchecked, could have led to "unwanted issues." Phew, close call!

Composed of the muscles of the lower abdomen, lower back, buttocks, and pelvic floor, it is the deep core muscles that support your spine and act as a natural corset (looks good, functions better). Core-oriented disciplines such as yoga, dance, Pilates, and martial arts all promote strengthening muscles in the midsection of the body to stabilize the spine and improve posture. So, which muscles belong to the "core"? It seems to depend on whom you ask, but I like to think of the "core" (or "powerhouse" in Pilates speak) as the key players in stabilizing the abdomen and spine.

**Breathing Diaphragm:** The breathing diaphragm plays an important role in core stabilization. An umbrella-shaped muscle that moves up and down when you breathe, with an extensive network of fascial connections to the front, back, and sides of the rib cage, and to the spine. Not sure what I mean by "fascial connections"? You'll learn more about those later in this chapter (preview: they keep your muscles long and lean and may even help with cellulite!).

**Pelvic Floor:** This consists of a collection of muscles that stretch across the base of the pelvis. If you put your hands on your hips and imagine that your hands are on the top edges of a bowl, you can imagine your pelvic floor as the bottom of the bowl. Your pelvic floor, as the name suggests, supports your pelvic organs including your bladder, urethra, uterus, vagina, and rectum. When the pelvic floor muscles contract, they contract inward and upward, supporting pelvic organs and also squeezing around the urethra, vagina, and rectum. In addition to holding your organs in place, these muscles serve as a closing mechanism.

**Transverse Abdominis (TVA):** This is the deepest abdominal muscle, wrapping around you from either side of your spine like a corset. The TVA moves in and out, and when posture and alignment are in the correct form, it works with the pelvic floor muscles.

**Multifidus:** These are the short muscles that extend out from both sides of your spine, starting at your tailbone (sacrum) and going all the way up to your neck. Their purpose is to support and protect your spine, and work together with the TVA and pelvic floor muscles to stabilize and support the low back and pelvis both before, and during, movement. If your multifidus muscles are weak, it can lead to low back pain. Pain can also reduce the function of these muscles, creating an unfortunate pain-weakness cycle.

While we are on the subject of core strength, I want you to take a moment to contemplate your navel. More precisely, bring your focus to the space around your navel, the area of the solar plexus, and up to the breastbone. This area, known as the *Manipura* or "third" chakra, governs self-esteem, warrior energy, and transformation. If you're associating chakras with rainbows and unicorns, you're partially right, but only about the rainbow part. Chakras are concentrated centers of energy located up the midline of the body, from the base of the spine to the top of the head, and each chakra is associated with an element, a color (there's your rainbow), and an area of the body. You'll learn way more about this in the following chapter! When the seven chakra centers are open, healthy, and flowing, that life-force energy contributes to our well-being in a powerful way. Manipura is literally at the core of who we are. The abdomen and lower thoracic/lumbar spine are the body parts associated with this chakra, and it is where we hold self-acceptance, self-respect, and our personal power. When this chakra is blocked, we can feel a lot of body shame and insecurity, and experience difficulty following through with changes we wish to cultivate in our lives. Developing core strength and awareness is your secret weapon in achieving balance—not only physically, but on an energetic level—to cultivate real change in your life.

## Consistency Counts. A Lot.

Our bodies were made for movement. Movement shapes our muscles, strengthens our heart, and elevates our mood. It increases our intake of oxygen, providing energy for our cells, muscles, ligaments, tendons, and organs. Movement also stimulates blood flow to help us utilize the nutrients we put into our bodies, enhancing digestion, absorption, and elimination. The load that we put on our bones and joints during exercise helps us maintain bone density, and we need that not only for moving our bodies, but to protect our brain, heart, and other organs from injury. When I learned that we achieve peak bone mass in our twenties and that loss of bone density can start as early as age thirty-five, I was grateful that I found movement early in life and that I'd remained consistent over the years. Natural movements like walking, squatting, kneeling, lifting, and even changing positions throughout the day are key to overall wellness. In his recently published book *The New Health Rules*, Dr. Frank Lipman writes that we tend to fall into one camp or the other when it comes to fitness—"go-go power exercisers or chill yoga loyalists"—and that the truth is, we need balance. If you live mostly in column A, grab something from column B once a week, and vice versa. He also suggests we regularly throw in a good stretch session after intense lifting at the gym and that we pay more attention to our core. His advice to "one way or another, do something physical every single day" is very much in line with my own fitness philosophy.

I like to move in a variety of ways and my body loves that too. That high-intensity interval training (HIIT) I mentioned? It only takes 20 minutes, twice a week, and studies have found that HIIT releases human growth hormone (HGH). This magical hormone that keeps you lean, energized, and feeling sexy begins to drop dramatically around age thirty, so the longer you can keep your body producing HGH, the better! Along with HIIT, I find TRX classes to be an amazing way to gain strength using your own body weight, and functional training with weights improves balance, strength, and endurance. While I like to switch things up, both Pilates and yoga remain a constant in my life. They are both transformational, focused methods of movement that facilitate positive change in the body, mind, and spirit (you know I'm all about that!). Rotating core strength practice with a well-rounded asana practice is a perfect way to strike the right balance. The expansive stretching achieved in yoga provides great range of motion and a wonderful balance to core-oriented Pilates exercises. The core strength and muscle integration you develop in Pilates will give you the stability you need to control your movements and safely expand into more challenging yoga poses. Regardless of what is on my movement menu for the day, I *always* make time for my foam roller and spend a few minutes bouncing about on my rebounder, which aside from providing detox benefits, is a fantastic way to strengthen your pelvic floor (and avoid "unwanted issues"!).

## Our Issues Are in Our Tissues

If you're familiar with the popular saying "our issues are in our tissues," a more precise way to describe this concept might be "our issues are in our fascia." I learned this firsthand during my recovery from spinal surgery, when I was fortunate enough to work with a physical therapist that introduced me to the miracle that is our fascia system. I've often been curious about the connection between

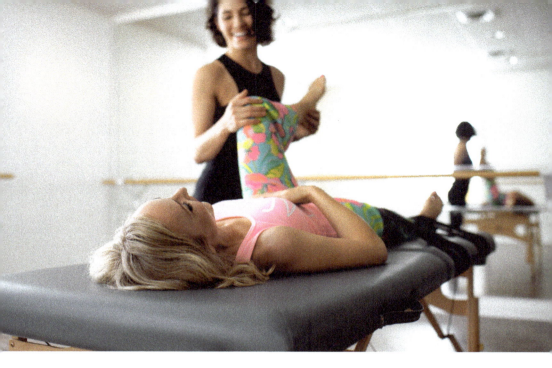

receiving bodywork and having old, unprocessed emotions come up for me, or how releasing tension in one area of my body seemed to relax other areas of my body as well. Turns out the answer to both of these questions lies within our fascia—the largest and richest sensory organ in the human body that you've likely never heard of.

Fascia (pronounced FASH-ya) is a thick layer of connective tissue that encases your entire body under your skin, wrapping itself around every muscle, joint, and organ. Under a microscope, fascia is a highly organized mesh of tubules filled with water. Its job is to attach, stabilize, enclose, and separate the muscles and internal organs. Fascia is largely responsible for the shape of your body, as well as the health and function of your muscles, joints, arteries, veins, brain, and spinal cord. In its healthy state, fascia is smooth, supple, and slides easily. This allows you to move and stretch to your full length in any direction. All fascia is connected, so what happens in one area of the body, for better or worse, actually affects the fascia in all areas of the body. If you feel stiff, inflexible, or off balance, there's a good chance your fascia has developed adhesions, or tight places where tissues that should be separated by fascia have been fused. Injury can create adhesions, as can inflammation, chronic stress, and unprocessed emotions.

# Fascia Release

There are numerous ways to address dense fascia, including yoga, Pilates, and acupuncture, as well as various forms of bodywork such as Rolfing, Yamuna ball rolling, and Fascial Stretch Therapy (FST). You can find some good introductory videos on most of these techniques on YouTube. My favorite way to work my fascia on my own is by using a foam roller. The roller delves into the fascia in much the same way bodywork does, improving blood circulation throughout fascia, skin, muscles, and joints. It's helpful to work with a professional who can assist you in developing a routine that addresses your specific needs and can coach you around your form, but here are a few basics to get you started:

**Snow Angels**

- Place the foam roller vertically and lie on it so that the base of your head and the bottom of your spine sit comfortably on the roller, knees bent about hips' width apart. Begin with your arms extended down by your sides, with the palms of your hands facing up to open and expand the chest. Hang out here for a bit and notice your body relaxing into the foam as you take a few slow deep breaths (that part is pretty awesome). When you feel ready, inhale deeply as you reach your arms up overhead slowly and with control, keeping them as close to the mat as possible and parallel to the floor. Exhale completely as you draw your arms back down to the sides. Repeat this movement eight to ten times.

**Diaphragm Release**

- Place the foam roller underneath the bottom of your shoulder blades and gently interlace your fingers, placing them behind your head to support your neck. Place your feet on the floor, knees bent and feet hip-width apart. Slowly inhale as you arch your middle back over the roller and slowly exhale as you curl back (as if you were performing a crunch), squeezing all the air out of your belly. Repeat this movement eight to ten times.

**IT Band Stretch**

- Lie on your side and place the foam roller just beneath the big bony structure of your hip. Keeping your arms straight, or bent for modification, slowly roll the foam down the side of your leg, stopping just above your knee joint. Be mindful not to cross the knee joint, as this can cause irritation in that sensitive area. Repeat this movement slowly (about 8 seconds for each roll) and perform three or four times on each side.

So much of our physical state is a result of the stress and tension we carry around with us on a day-to-day basis, and many of us carry the extra burden of unresolved emotions with us as well. Our body and spirit are made up of energy, and energy must be allowed to flow to stay vital and clear. You may find that emotions, memories, and thoughts stored in your fascia come up as you begin moving your body. That's okay! In fact that's awesome, because allowing your old thoughts and feelings to come up and flow through you releases them from your tissue. This release activates your body's self-healing process and deepens your mind-body connection, allowing you to really listen, inhabit, and care for your body.

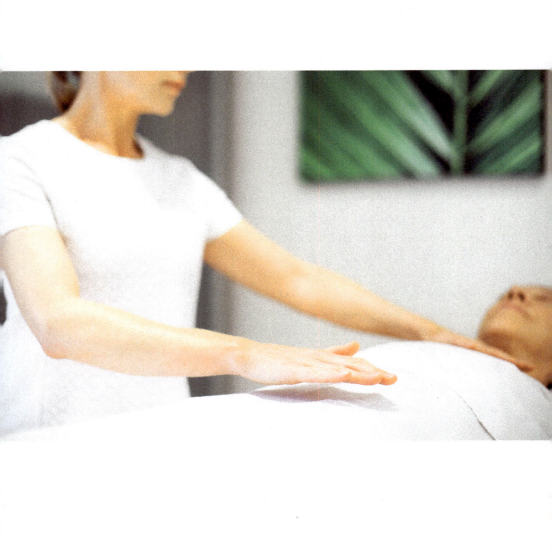

# Chapter Four
# What Is This Woo-Woo Stuff? (The Part Where I Talk about Your Chakras)

## Are You Breathing, Honey?

**My Mama Ruth** used to ask me this question a lot and honestly, it annoyed me. It annoyed me because of course she was right, I wasn't breathing, but also because it meant that I had to deal with my shit. Sometimes I just wanted to hide out in my non-breathing state so that I could numb myself to whatever unpleasant situation happened to be occurring for me in that moment. I mean this literally. Go ahead and hold your breath and you'll see what I mean. Holding your breath numbs you both physically and emotionally, but you can't continue to hold your breath forever. Eventually you will have to breathe, and when you do, you will find yourself right back in your body. And when you arrive back in your body your feelings will still be there, because here's the truth about the things we don't want to look at: they tend to stick around. They hang out, waiting for you to acknowledge them, and they have *a lot* of patience. They will wait for you to do your whole avoidance thing—they don't mind. In fact, your avoidance is like superfood for unacknowledged feelings; it makes them grow bigger and stronger, sometimes entirely unrecognizable in their new form. In this super state, our feelings can act out in ways that keep us further from our truths, further from the life we envision for ourselves, and further from the vibrant health we all deserve.

Experiencing a full range of emotions is a vital part of our human experience and a marker of true health. It took decades for me to allow this simple truth to sink into my being. For me to feel, on a cellular level, safe enough to feel everything (even the shameful, icky things). I struggled with body image, denied myself pleasure, and sought out the comfort of numbness, all in an effort to escape the very thing that would bring about the healing I longed for: *experiencing* my feelings. Keeping myself stuck in my disordered eating seemed *way* easier than facing the things in my life that I created an eating disorder to avoid in the first place. When that distraction wasn't enough, drugs and alcohol provided a welcome, if temporary, sense of relief. Unfortunately, no amount of numbing takes the pain of our difficult life experiences away. In fact, the numbing can act as the perfect fuel to keep the pain alive inside you, allowing it to remain a part of your present experience. My father used alcohol and heroin to keep his truths from coming in, but his addictions just fed those truths until they were all that existed. That's a lot of precious life to give away! We are all so much more than our pain. We are our joy, our compassion, our love. What if we fed those aspects of ourselves? And what if in doing so, we created the perfect environment for not just healing, but *thriving* in our lives? What could that look like for you?

## Your Spirit's Unfinished Business

> *"Your soul is rooting for you."*
> — Danielle LaPorte #truthbomb

When unprocessed emotions from our life experiences live in our bodies, we may feel them at some level all the time. You might recognize them as that pit in your stomach, fluttering in your chest, or tears that spring to your eyes when you recall a certain event, and this is an indication that the energy around it remains lodged in your body. Remember, emotions (energy in motion = e-motion) are meant to flow through us so that we can experience them, not hold on to them. Energy that has been trapped in the body—whether from trauma, heartbreak, grief, or other difficult emotions—needs a vehicle for release. I like to think of this energy as my spirit's unfinished business, and my very own body as the perfect vehicle for allowing this release to (gently) occur. Maybe your spirit has unfinished business too.

## You're in Your Feelings & Some of Them Suck—Now What?

In previous chapters you had the opportunity to get clear on where you are, how you feel, and to consider how you might like to feel different. What happens when you allow yourself the space to become more aware of how you feel both physically and emotionally? Sometimes it can be like lifting a fog, allowing more clarity and light into your life. Clarity and light are good … and sometimes scary (it's okay to have both). Now, back to that feelings part. When you begin to feel your feelings, some of them might very well suck, but that's not the worst thing ever. Those feelings are offerings from your body, little clues from your soul, letting you know what in your life might want your attention. What you do with that offering is *your* choice. Your soul will root for you anyway, because that's just what it does.

The tools you will be given in this chapter will help you begin to notice where in your body you are holding on to things that keep you stuck; and shift your thoughts about where you are, right here and now. By shifting your thinking, it's way easier to instinctively make choices that support you on your journey. Know that the action of simply *noticing* where you are is an act of courageous self-care, and the fact that you are willing to notice means you are awesome!

## The Part Where I Talk about Your Chakras

Growing up in the Northern California coastal community of Bodega, it was pretty much mandatory to have a working knowledge of the Chakra system (and yes, there may have been a healing crystal or two in my home). Long before I integrated energy medicine into my health coaching practice, I used it as part of my daily self-care regime. One of the things I love about energy medicine is that it's so readily available for each of us to use, any time we want. You don't have to be a trained practitioner to have the personal experience of sensing—and shifting—the energy in your body. We have within us the innate ability to heal, on all the levels we are. Energy medicine is a terrific way for us to harness that ability to create balance in the body.

## What Is This Woo-Woo Stuff?

> *"In every culture and in every medical tradition before ours, healing was accomplished by moving energy."*
> — Albert Szent-Györgyi, Biochemist and Nobel Prize Winner

The term "energy medicine" became popular in the 1980s, but working with our energies to promote health is in no way a new concept. The knowledge that an unseen energy flows through all living things and directly affects the quality of our physical, mental, and spiritual health has been a part of the wisdom of many cultures throughout history. The concept of life-force energy is found in most ancient cultures in the world. In India, it's called prana; in China, chi; in Japan, ki; and for Native Americans, the Great Spirit. There are many different types of energy medicine, some being traced back to ancient healing traditions such as acupuncture, Qigong, and yoga. Energy medicine employs diverse methods to work with the flow of energy within the body, with the intent to realign, replenish, or stabilize the amount and quality of energy. It is both a complement to other approaches to health care, and a complete system for self-care. It can address physical, emotional, or mental imbalances, as well as support your body's immune system and ability to heal.

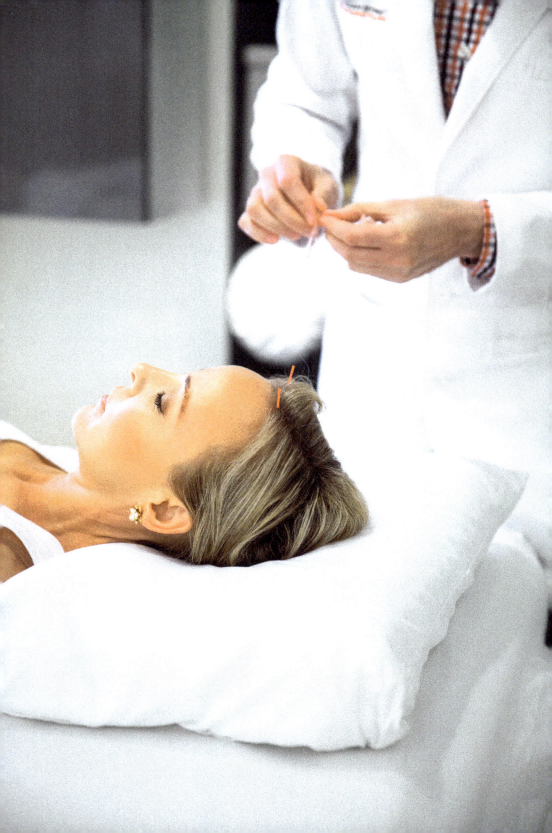

# How I Use Energy Medicine (and How *You* Can Too!)

I take a pretty loose, intuitive approach to how I use energy medicine. While I have a working knowledge of a variety of energy practices, I believe that each of us carries this knowledge within us and that the study of energy medicine provides an opportunity to tap into what our miraculous bodies already know. I first recognized this when I was introduced to a Qigong exercise called "Cleanse the Qi"—a practice of gathering the calm energy around you, washing it through your entire body, and then sending it down and out through your feet. The movement of the practice felt comforting and familiar, as if it were a part of my own body. Then I realized I had instinctively been doing this since I was a child! Whenever I experienced a situation where the energy of a room (or the people in it) felt out of alignment with my own, I would do a "cleansing" and feel much more at home in my body. Who knows, you might have a similar experience as you discover a variety of ways to work with your own energy throughout this chapter!

While I believe each of us has the innate ability to work with our own energy to create balance and health in the body, there are benefits to developing a more "formal" energy practice. For instance, there are subtle variations in posture, breathing, and even eye gaze that enhance the effects of energy medicine. The Qigong practice "Cleanse the Qi" is performed in something called "wuji" posture, which is the foundation of all dynamic (moving) and quiescent (static) standing exercises. This posture maximizes both relaxation and the flow of qi. While the posture may be intuitive, tightening your anal sphincter or touching your tongue to the upper palate behind your teeth to seal in the qi and prevent it from leaking may not be.

While the study of energy medicine is endlessly fascinating to me and I consider my practice an essential part of my daily routine, I don't always have a ton of time to dedicate to it. This is where having a working knowledge of a variety of practices comes in handy, because regardless of whether I have five minutes or an hour, I still get awesome benefits. Here's what that looks like for me, and what it can look like for *you* too:

**I Breathe:** Sometimes this is as simple as taking a long, deep breath when I notice my breathing is shallow (yes, I still hold my breath!). Other times I get pretty specific about my intention for breath work and have some go-to protocols that I'm excited to share with you. If the other energy practices I'm presenting here are simply too woo-woo for you, no worries. Feel free to just breathe (you have to anyway) and see if all that breathing opens you up for more!

**I Go to Acupuncture:** I'm a huge fan of acupuncture and have found treatments to be immensely helpful for a variety of issues (hormonal imbalance, chronic pain, anxiety, depression, and allergies to name a few). My perfect week definitely includes a session with needles, but perfect doesn't always happen. While experiencing acupuncture for yourself requires an appointment and I hope you make one, practicing *acupressure* on yourself does not.

**I Practice Reiki:** I practice Reiki on myself, family, friends, clients, and even my dog! My Aunt Patty introduced Reiki to me when I was just a kid, so the concept of hands-on healing is second nature to me. Over the years I continued to feel drawn to its gentle, healing ways, so I decided to learn it myself. Now I get to experience Reiki any time I want and you can too. I'll be telling you exactly how in a later chapter.

**I Practice Yoga:** As a kid, time on my mat meant time with Mama Ruth (and her *Yoga for Health* record). I loved just about anything if it involved hanging out with my mama, so I quickly loved yoga and I still do. I especially love to practice Kundalini yoga with internationally celebrated husband and wife team Ana Brett and Ravi Singh. While they travel extensively teaching workshops, conferences, and retreats worldwide, I can practice with them any time I want and you can too. I've been collecting their DVDs for the better part of a decade, and they now offer yoga streams on their website, lovetribevibes.com. If practicing on your own isn't your thing, the app "Om Finder" can help you find classes at nearly 7,000 studios in 63 countries worldwide and can be filtered by time and type. In his book *The*

*New Health Rules*, Dr. Frank Lipman writes that yoga is about a lot of things, but largely it's about learning how to stay in an uncomfortable place and that you can take that anywhere you want … to your work life, to relationships, to parenting, to finances. The concept goes wherever you need it. In this way, yoga changes everything.

**I Practice Qigong (pronounced "chee gong"):** Qigong is considered a collective term for a long-established, extensive set of exercises first created in China more than 2,000 years ago. It involves performing gentle movements that are synchronized with the inhalations and exhalations of the breath, making it similar to yoga. The word "qi" translates literally to life force, and "gong" means the practice of developing more qi or life-force energy. I'll be introducing you to a fun way to experience your own life-force energy through the practice of Qigong in this chapter.

**I Balance My Chakras:** Between my yoga practice, breath work, and meditations, I've got my chakras pretty well covered, but I do carry crystals in my pockets for good measure (yes, really).

**I Practice EFT Tapping:** Tapping just might be my favorite thing ever! The Emotional Freedom Technique (EFT for short) is a powerful yet simple method of energetic healing that works directly with the meridian system used in Traditional Chinese Medicine (TCM). I used it for the first time to sort out my driving anxiety, and after a few short sessions, I was able to transform my fears and get my driver's license for the first time at age forty-six! I was blown away by how immediate and effective EFT was, and I continue to use it to treat a variety of issues on my own and with my clients. In the following chapter you'll have the opportunity to try Tapping for yourself … prepare to be amazed!

**I Hug Trees:** You may have guessed this already, but I'm a total tree hugger! While I do literally hug trees given the opportunity, research has shown that you don't even have to touch a tree to experience its healing benefits; you simply need to be within its vicinity. While this isn't news to the large groups of people practicing tai chi in city parks, the health-promoting properties of trees has been validated by science. In his book *Blinded by Science*, Matthew Silverstone explains that it's the vibrational properties of trees and plants that offer health benefits, not just open space. When one touches a tree, its different vibrational pattern will affect various biological behaviors within the body. Taoist master Mantak Chia teaches how to align one's body with the energetic field of a tree and explains that trees are natural processors that can help you transform your body's negative energy into positive, vital life-force energy. As you connect your energy with the tree, you facilitate your own physical and emotional healing. Go get yourself out in the world and hug a tree, exercise in nature, or simply smile at a tree next time you see one. Your energy will thank you for it!

**I Believe in Flower Power:** When I was growing up, Mama Ruth kept a wooden box full of tiny vials of the original Bach Flower Remedies. Mysterious and magical, these little tinctures of flower essence got us through some tricky times. I didn't think much about how or why, but I sure found comfort in Mama reading from the list of Bach Flower Remedies and their indications. I liked to look over the list of 38 individual flower essences and intuitively pick one for Mama Ruth to read aloud:

> **Aspen:** "Vague unknown fears for which there can be given no explanation, no reason. It is a terror that something awful is going to happen even though it is unclear what exactly. These vague inexplicable fears may haunt by night or day. Sufferers may often be afraid to tell their trouble to others." — Dr. Edward Bach
>
> **Indication:** Fears and worries of unknown origin.

We would continue on with our ritual of picking remedies and reading their indications until I felt we had all my bases covered. Looking back, that ritual was not only wonderful because Mama Ruth was mixing up just the right tincture to soothe me, she was also teaching me to identify my feelings (a worthwhile endeavor on its own). I was also learning that I was not alone in my feelings, whatever my feelings happened to be. More recently, I got curious about what was happening and why it always seemed to help. Here's what I learned: Flower alchemy is the practice of harnessing the life-force energy of a plant, which can be captured in a water and alcohol solution. When taken internally or applied externally, this energy works through the acupuncture meridians to shift our state of mind. This shift occurs within minutes, with a growing effect over time. A simple way to experience this shift yourself is to grab a bottle of the popular "Rescue Remedy" (readily available at your local health food store or online) so that you have it on hand when you need it. This mix of Impatiens, Star of Bethlehem, Cherry Plum, Rock Rose, and Clematis was created by Dr. Bach to deal with emergencies and crises. It's perfect for that moment when there is no time to make a proper individual selection of remedies, but you're super stressed and want relief fast.

**I Read Books:** Specifically, I love to read books like this:

- *The Subtle Body: An Encyclopedia of Your Energetic Anatomy* by Cyndi Dale because, well, it's *everything*. It deeply explores the chakras, energy meridians, acupuncture, reflexology, Ayurveda, Qigong, Kabbalah, and so much more. It's an amazing resource for understanding the physical, energetic, and spiritual elements of health.

- Anything by Donna Eden because she's been teaching people how to work with the body's energy systems for more than three decades! She's a wealth of knowledge, and her books have handy routines for both general balancing and a wide variety of specific ailments. *The Little Book of Energy Medicine* is one of my favorites.

- *Reiki: A Comprehensive Guide* by Pamela Miles (forward by Donna Eden) truly is a comprehensive guide. I think I bought the book because it had Donna Eden's "seal of approval," but I read it cover to cover and then made the decision to formally offer Reiki to my clients. If you're interested in learning more about Reiki, this is your book.

- *Heal Yourself with Qigong* by Suzanne B. Friedman, LAC, is an awesome book not only because it presents over 100 easy five-minute Qigong exercises designed to target a wide variety of specific health issues, but it also gives you a chance to do a deep dive into everything Qigong if that interests you. Suzanne Friedman is an acupuncturist, herbalist, and doctor of medical qigong therapy who chairs the Medical Qigong Science Department at the Acupuncture and Integrative Medicine College in Berkeley, CA (she knows her stuff!).

- *Acupressure's Potent Points: A Guide to Self-Care for Common Ailments* by Michael Reed Gach was loaned to me by my physical therapist, Patrick Bridgett. Patrick was instrumental to my recovery following spinal surgery not only because he's a gifted PT, but also because he's a generous and compassionate human being with a wealth of knowledge about the body and its amazing ability to heal. Weekly appointments with Patrick for more than a year taught me many things (a lot of them involving a foam roller), but the most important thing I learned was how to play the starring role in my own healing. I'm forever grateful for the wisdom he shared with me. I'm also grateful for the many books he was kind enough to lend me (this one I never gave back).

- *The Tapping Solution: A Revolutionary System for Stress-Free Living* by Nick Ortner was my first introduction to the world of Tapping, and to say that it transformed my life is an understatement. This book can help you examine what's holding you back in literally *any* area of your life, but more importantly, Nick shows you how you can use this profound practice to let go of patterns that no longer serve you and live your happiest, healthiest life.

## Your (Brief) Energy Anatomy Lesson

Meridians, chakras, aura, basic grid, Celtic weave, five rhythms, triple warmer, radiant circuits, and the electrics ... oh my! The study of energy medicine is an exhaustive and complex endeavor—one worthy of books dedicated to a deep dive of the systems that form our intricate energy anatomy, of which there are many. This is not one of those books, but I do have some favorites in my personal library and they are listed above. For our purposes here, the following is your (brief) energy anatomy lesson:

**Meridians:** The meridians are energy pathways (I like to imagine tiny rivers) for chi—the foundation of Traditional Chinese Medicine (TCM). In the same way that an artery transports blood, a meridian transports life-force energy (chi). Acupuncturists work with these meridians to stimulate and encourage the smooth flow of chi and blood throughout the body, which also triggers the body's own healing mechanism. Meridian pathways bring energy to the immune, nervous, endocrine, circulatory, respiratory, digestive, skeletal, muscular, and lymphatic systems. Though traditional Eastern medicine has had a successful run for *thousands* of years, science had yet to confirm the existence of meridians until now. Scientists at Seoul National University injected a special staining dye onto acupuncture points, allowing them to see thin lines. These same lines were not visible at non-acupuncture sites where there are no meridians. They believe this discovery is in fact the physical component of the Acupuncture Meridian System, which they refer to as the "primo-vascular system." Previously, scientists had used a combination of imaging techniques and CT scans, allowing them to observe concentrated points of microvascular structures that correspond to the map of acupuncture points created by Chinese energy practitioners in ancient times.

**Acupuncture & Acupressure Points:** Acupuncture works by stimulating specific points on the surface of your skin called "acupuncture points." These points are pools of accumulated energy located on the meridians that run throughout the body, with high concentrations of nerve endings, mast cells, lymphatics, and capillaries—all capable of triggering biochemical and physiological changes in the body. Acupuncture (with needles) and acupressure (with fingers) use the same points and meridians.

**Chakras:** The chakras are concentrated centers of energy located up the midline of the body from the base of the spine to the top of the head. There are seven chakras, which are believed to energetically record every emotionally significant event that you experience. Cyndi Dale, the author of *The Subtle Body: An Encyclopedia of Your Energetic Anatomy*, refers to the chakras as the power centers that run the "you inside of you" (I like that). These energy centers connect our nerves, hormones, and emotions. Their locations run parallel to the body's neuroendocrine-immune system and form a link between our vibrational anatomy and our physical anatomy. Though Western medicine has not recognized chakras yet, Eastern cultures have long appreciated them. Whether you perceive chakras as literal places in the body or as metaphoric ones, they can help you activate mind-body connections to help you heal.

**The Aura:** The aura is a multilayered protective sphere of energy that interacts with the energies within you and the atmosphere around you. Scientists who have detected the aura's energy call it the "biofield." If you are interested in seeing what *your* aura looks like on any given day, you're in luck. Aura photography is a thing (a one-of-a kind, palm-sized Polaroid kind of thing). Russian electrical engineer Semyon Kirlian invented the process in the 1930s, and in the 1970s Guy Coggins built a camera that can actually capture the human biofield. Christina Lonsdale of Radiant Human got her hands on one of these magical cameras (there are supposedly 100 of them) and she takes it on the road (literally). Radiant Human is a roving aura photography laboratory that could be touring in your city (they announce tour plans on Instagram @radianthuman_).

### Breathe. Exhale. Repeat.

Breath-focused meditation allows you to become more aware of your breath, and as you begin to work with it consciously, you create a direct link to a part of yourself that usually functions outside of conscious awareness. Taking time to observe your breath can be immensely helpful in managing your emotions and nonjudgmentally addressing your painful experiences. Ideally, we are present enough to our feelings to actually work through them in real time, as they are happening. Doing this keeps everything in perspective. Of course, ideal doesn't always happen, so we start where we are and we breathe.

### Breathing into *You*

- Begin to pay attention to your breath, watching your inhales and exhales as they come and go.
- Allow yourself to become curious about the depth and pace of your breathing. What would it feel like to lengthen your inhales and exhales?
- What if you paused at the top of your inhale for just a second or two, and again at the bottom of your exhale?
- Allow your face, neck, shoulders, and back to be easy. Allow your hips, legs, and feet to be easy as well. If you feel discomfort in any area of your body, dedicate the next inhale and exhale to it.
- Continue to breathe in this space for ten more long, deep breaths.
- When you are ready, gently open your eyes. Not ready? Just go ahead and breathe for as long as it takes!

Next time you find yourself holding your breath or needing to plant yourself back into that lovely body of yours, you would be wise to follow Mama Ruth's advice and breathe, honey! Let's practice it now so that you are more likely to remember it when you really need it.

### Long, Deep Breathing

This seemingly simple breath is an amazing method for moving energy and is the basic breath used in Kundalini yoga. Long Deep Breathing uses the full capacity of the lungs—something most of us rarely (if ever) do. It starts by filling the abdomen, then expanding the chest, and finally lifting the upper ribs and clavicle. The exhale is in the reverse: the collarbone deflates, then the chest, and finally the abdomen pulls in and up, as the navel pulls back toward the spine. Each part of the breath expansion is distinct, and when all three are combined you have a complete Long Deep Breath.

I find it helpful to learn this breath in three parts, because it gives you an opportunity to really notice where your breath is in your body. To begin, you can sit either on the floor or in a chair. If you are on the floor, grab a pillow or blanket if that's comfy for you. Sit up straight and place your left hand on your belly, your right hand on your chest. Okay, let's breathe!

**Part I: Abdominal Breath**

- Bring your attention to your navel and take a slow, deep breath by letting the belly relax and expand.

- As you exhale, gently pull the navel in and up toward the spine. This pushing allows a portion of the lower lungs to be used efficiently.

- Keep your chest relaxed and focus on breathing entirely with the lower abdomen. On your inhale, notice the expansion of your belly and monitor the chest with your other hand—it should remain still and relaxed.

**Part II: Chest Breath**

- Using the chest muscles, inhale slowly, focusing on the sensation of expansion and keeping the diaphragm still. Exhale completely, but do not use the abdomen.

- Continue on for a few more rounds, comparing the depth and volume of this breath with the isolated abdominal breath. This breath is where many of us hang out all day, and it means that we aren't using the full capacity of our lungs.

**Part III: Clavicular Breath**

- Sit up straight and contract the navel in, keeping the abdomen tight. Lift the chest without inhaling. Now, inhale slowly by expanding the shoulders and collarbone. Really try to feel as if you are breathing in through your collarbone.

- If this one feels difficult for you, that's actually a good sign! If this is your normal breath, you are depriving yourself of life-giving oxygen. If you've ever watched a baby breathe, you will notice that it's naturally performing a long, deep breath. This means that you do already know how to breathe, you just forgot somewhere along your life … it happens.

**Putting It All Together: Long Deep Breath**

- Begin the inhale with an Abdominal Breath. Then add the Chest Breath and finish with a Clavical Breath. All three breaths are done in a smooth motion.

- Start the exhale by relaxing the clavicle, then slowly emptying the chest, and finally pull in the abdomen to force out any remaining air.

- Feels amazing, right? Keep breathing for another few Long Deep Breaths.

# Qigong: Developing Energy Awareness

> *"Simply put, everything vibrates, absolutely everything, from the nucleus of an atom to the molecules of our blood, our organs, our brain, light, sound, plants, animals, earth, space, the universe; they all have one thing in common—they all vibrate. This fundamental principle should be the basis of all science as it is the one principle that unifies everything, and if you can understand vibrations, everything else becomes clear."*
>
> — Matthew Silverstone, *Blinded by Science*

These simple exercises are a fun and easy way to develop an awareness of energy. Before beginning this exercise, take several long deep breaths to settle into your body. When you are finished, simply set an intention of feeling your life-force energy.

**Exercise 1: Creating the Ball of Energy**

- **Rub your hands together:** Do this briskly as if you were warming your hands together on a chilly day.
- **Intention:** Hold the intention of bringing, and feeling, your life-force energy into your hands.
- **Awareness:** Bring your awareness into your hands and feel for this life-force energy in each hand. Begin to notice the connection of energy between your two hands.
- **Pull your hands apart:** After your hands feel that they are filled with warmth and qi (your life-force energy), and that the connection between your two hands is strong, begin to pull them apart gently and slowly. Keep your hands and fingers soft and fluid, letting them flow smoothly through the air.
- **Bring your hands closer together:** When you feel the connection between your hands weaken, bring them back together slowly, but don't let them touch. Repeat this process of slowly moving your hands apart and then back together, maintaining a slow and steady rhythm. Feel the energy in your hands as well as the energy connecting them. See if you notice any changes in these energies as you complete the exercise.
- **To end:** At the end of this exercise, simply pull your hands apart slowly and let them drop at your sides. After you've mastered the basic energy ball exercise, continue on to the next exercise.

If you went through this exercise and have no idea if anything in particular happened for you, that's okay! Your body may simply go through the motions at first, but with a bit of practice, you're likely to notice a sensation between your palms. Some people feel this as heat, while others describe it as the force between two repelling magnets. Your own life force will feel unique to you!

**Exercise 2: Rotating the Energy Ball**

For this exercise, you want to begin by creating and feeling the energy between your hands like you did in the first exercise. When you are ready, move on to rotating the energy ball like this:

- Now that you've created your energy ball, keep your hands a constant distance apart. Slowly move them so one hand is on the top and the other is on the bottom. Or, one can move forward while the other moves back toward you, but always maintain the same distance between the hands.
- Continue moving the energy ball.

**Exercise 3: Shrinking, Growing, and Rotating the Energy Ball**

For this exercise, you will be combining exercises one and two and then adding a third element.

- Create and feel the energy between your hands.
- Keeping the connection between your hands, move them slowly apart and then back toward each other.
- At the same time, rotate your hands. You will be pulling and shrinking the energy ball from different directions.

## Chakras + Crystals

Belief in the power of healing stones dates back thousands of years to the earliest civilizations, and it's definitely having a moment in our current culture (not *just* my hippie friends). These days, you can purchase a "GOOP exclusive" pouch of magically charged

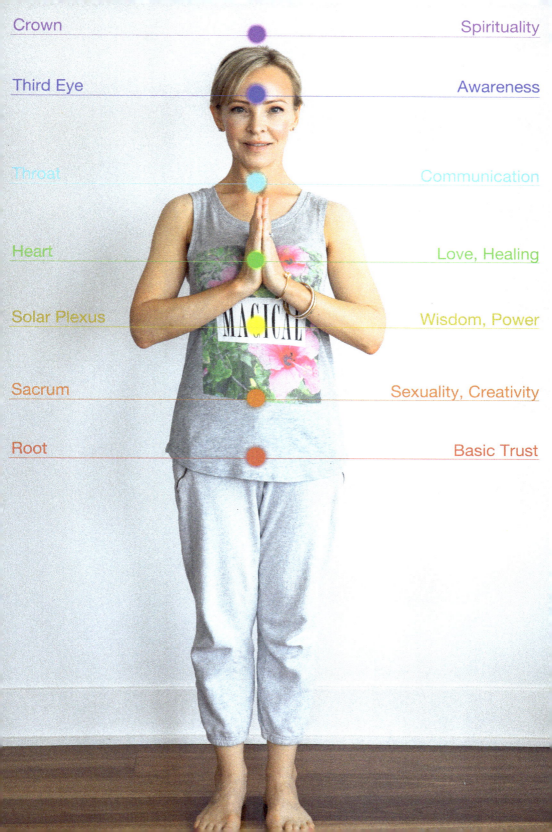

stones, enjoy sapphires and biotechnology from the Själ skincare line, while London's Nectar Café boasts a bottled "high-vibe hydration" crystal-infused water. Indeed, crystals are trending in a modern way! Using stones to balance your chakras is a pretty simple (and just plain pretty) way to incorporate energy medicine into your daily life.

### First or Root Chakra (red)

**You Feel:** fearful, ungrounded, and resistant to change

**You Want to Feel:** grounded and stable

**Healing Stones:** clear quartz, hematite, red jasper

### Second or Sacral Chakra (orange)

**You Feel:** overly sensitive or emotionally unbalanced

**You Want to Feel:** creative, emotionally balanced, and sexy

**Healing Stones:** clear quartz, carnelian, red jasper

### Third or Solar-Plexus Chakra (yellow)

**You Feel:** fearful or judgmental

**You Want to Feel:** grounded in your personal power

**Healing Stones:** clear quartz, amethyst, green moss agate, sapphire, scolecite

### Fourth or Heart Chakra (green/pink/gold)

**You Feel:** possessive or fearful of rejection

**You Want to Feel:** unconditional love and compassion

**Healing Stones:** clear quartz, green moss agate, rose quartz, sapphire, scolecite

### Fifth or Throat Chakra (blue/turquoise)

**You Feel:** unable to verbalize your needs, desires, and opinions

**You Want to Feel:** truthful in your verbal expression

**Healing Stones:** clear quartz, sapphire

### Sixth or Brow Chakra (indigo)

**You Feel:** uninspired and judgmental

**You Want to Feel:** focused, centered, and intuitive

**Healing Stones:** clear quartz, amethyst, green moss agate, sapphire, scolecite

### Seventh or Crown Chakra (violet)

**You Feel:** exhausted and depressed

**You Want to Feel:** connected to your higher awareness

**Healing Stones:** clear quartz, amethyst, scolecite

**Purchasing Your Crystals:** You may already be familiar with a handful of common stones like rose quartz, amethyst, or jade, but if you've never walked into a showroom full of gemstones you might get overwhelmed! I suggest showing a salesperson the following list of "10 essentials" and asking them to show you what's what. They will likely be super helpful and give off awesome vibes because they hang out with healing stones all day long. Here's the list:

**Amethyst:** third-eye and crown chakras

**Carnelian:** sacral chakra

**Citrine:** solar-plexus chakra

**Clear Quartz:** all chakras, but particularly the crown

**Green Moss Agate:** heart and third-eye chakras

**Hematite:** root chakra

**Red Jasper:** root and sacral chakras

**Rose Quartz:** heart, solar-plexus, and sacral chakras

**Sapphire:** throat, third-eye, solar-plexus, and heart chakras

**Scolecite:** heart, third-eye, and crown chakras

Keep in mind that there are *many* stones to choose from, so think of these "10 essentials" as a starting point for your personal collection. You might resonate with certain stones or be attracted to them based on your personal needs. Pick what you are drawn to (or what's drawn to *you*) and you won't go wrong. If you're looking to buy just one single crystal, make it the clear quartz. Its colorlessness allows you to substitute it for any stone. You can also use this high-vibrational stone to amplify the energy of other stones you have.

**Preparing Your Stones:** The first thing you'll want to do when you bring your stones home is to clean them. The idea behind this is that the stones have taken on the energy of the many hands they've passed through on their journey into *your* hands. I mostly stick with the wet or dry method of cleansing stones with sea salt to absorb negative energy, which looks like this:

> **Wet:** Fill a glass or ceramic bowl about half full with water and sea salt. Avoid using a metal bowl, as it can react with certain stones. Let them rest anywhere between 1 and 24 hours.

**Dry:** Fill a glass bowl about halfway up and either bury your stones in the dry salt or let them rest on its surface for anywhere between several hours and several days.

When you're finished cleaning your stones, rinse them in pure water and wipe them with a soft cloth. Traditionally, the ritual of "charging" them with energy and intention is the next step, and there are different ways to approach this. The practice of burying your stones in dirt for a week, allowing them to cleanse and recharge with the earth, is pretty cool. If you are so inclined and have access to soil (a houseplant works), do that. I also like to leave my stones in a windowsill for 24 hours and let both the sun and moon work their magic. In the morning I take a few minutes to let them know my intention for working with them, and I'm good to go!

**Tip:** Your friends will likely be drawn to your new collection of sparkly gems and want to touch them. If someone else touches your crystals (so hard to resist), you'll want to clean them again before you use them. I'm not suggesting your friends have bad vibes, it's just that your crystals are now attuned to *your* vibes.

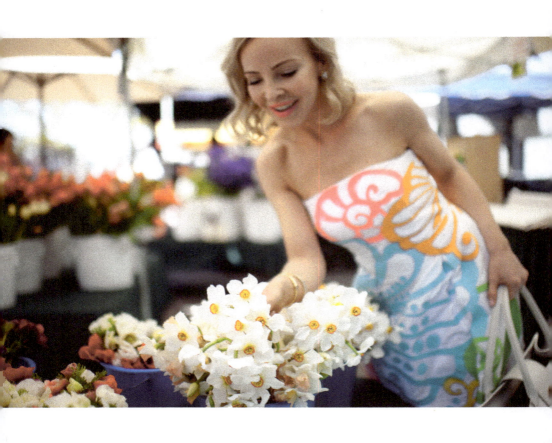

# Chapter Five
## Cultivating Pleasure
## (The Part Where I Talk about Orgasms)

*"What I want to encourage is the reclamation of the power of pleasure, which comes from the divine force of the universe. Pleasure is a divine gift to us. It should be a discipline practiced regularly to establish happiness and joy in your body and your life. Sustainable pleasure is the ultimate prescription for good health."*

— Dr. Christiane Northrup, *Goddesses Never Age*

**Pursuing pleasure, and** allowing ourselves to receive it on a regular basis, is essential to creating vibrant health and radiant beauty. When you immerse yourself in the joy of pleasure, you are renewing your cells and creating vibrant health on all the levels you are: body, mind, and spirit. Now, you may be wondering exactly what do I mean by "pleasure"? Am I talking orgasms here? Well yes (among other things), I am talking about the pleasure and health-boosting benefits of orgasm. After all, Dr. Christiane Northrup explains it so perfectly: "your body itself was conceived in orgasm and from that perspective, how could pleasure *not* play a vital role in the optimal functioning of your body?" Orgasms are just one opportunity out of limitless opportunities you have to experience pleasure in your life, and while you may believe cultivating pleasure is as simple as booking a mani pedi with your bestie or pouring a glass of wine, *sustainable* pleasure can be trickier than you think.

In this chapter we will explore how you can use activities like meditation, EFT Tapping, and (yes!) orgasms to both calm your nervous system *and* increase your pleasure. Calming your nervous system is key, because it's super hard to cultivate pleasure when you're stressed, even though it's *exactly* what you need. We'll also work on changing any limiting beliefs you may have accumulated on your life journey (it happens) so that they don't hold you back from experiencing all the pleasure you deserve. Some of the practices in this chapter are quick and easy, while others encourage you to set aside a period of time to lovingly care for the one and only you. The great thing is, they all work. So, pick what appeals to you or go wild and try them all!

## Your Brain on Pleasure: Yes, Please!

Cultivating pleasure is about learning to recognize the things that bring you lasting joy, and then deliberately bringing them into your life on a regular basis. It's also about nitric oxide. As it turns out, a tiny molecule produced in your very own body is the key to experiencing pleasure! Ferid Murad, MD, PhD, shared the 1998 Nobel Prize in Medicine for his research leading to the discovery that nitric oxide is your body's signaling molecule. With enough nitric oxide in your body, your blood vessel walls relax, allowing more oxygen and nutrients to flow to your heart, brain, and internal organs, supporting them in functioning optimally. Activities like acupuncture, massage, meditation, yoga, and sex have all been shown to stimulate the production of nitric oxide. Sufficient amounts of nitric oxide trigger more positive emotions like joy, resilience, and hope (more is more!). If you're a runner, you've likely experienced that sought-after "runners high," and that's nitric oxide at work. The sensation of nitric oxide being released lasts mere seconds, but it sets off a chain reaction of other feel-good chemicals in your body. On the flip side, if your levels are not high enough, your cells begin to break down, setting the stage for aches, pains, and chronic degenerative disease. Poor lifestyle choices such as eating the Standard American Diet (SAD), not moving your body enough, or smoking contribute to lower levels of nitric oxide, as can chronic stress and unprocessed emotions. Flooding your body with nitric oxide improves the health of your whole body and allows you to experience limitless amounts of pleasure ... yes, please!

## Your Brain on Stress: Fight. Flight. Freeze.

That life can be stressful is pretty much a given, but while stress is usually seen as a negative, it's important to understand that stress can be super helpful. We need the surge of chemicals to help us fight (defend ourselves), take flight (escape), or freeze (hide) to avoid danger. Here's how it works: when we experience a stressful situation, the hypothalamus secretes corticotrophin-releasing hormone to the pituitary, which then releases adrenocorticotropic hormone to the adrenal glands, which in turn releases cortisol. This chain of hormonal secretion is called the HPA axis and describes the three glands involved: the hypothalamus and the pituitary are single glands in the brain, and the adrenals are a pair, situated at the top of the kidneys. Given the traveling distance involved to signal a threat, if the HPA axis were the only alarm system we had to activate the fight-or-flight response, we'd be in trouble! That's where our sympathetic nervous system comes in to save the day (and your ass), by sending express signals from your brain to your nervous system and connecting everywhere from head to toes. This pattern helps us stay alive, which is obviously a good thing; it's what we *do* with that energy afterward that gets us into so much trouble.

Cortisol is a life-sustaining adrenal hormone essential to the maintenance of homeostasis, and while it serves many functions, in the fight-or-flight response, its job is to suppress the immune system. It does this because saving you from an immediate life-threatening danger takes precedence over fighting pathogens. When the sympathetic nervous system receives a danger signal, it increases heart rate, muscle response, blood pressure, and other systems to put you in a state of hyper-alarm. It also slows down or stops your digestion and sends blood from your stomach into your extremities, allowing you to either fight or take flight. After the perceived danger is over, the parasympathetic nervous system steps in and reverses the process, slowing everything down and speeding up digestion. Protect first, repair and nourish later.

## Phew, That's Over!

Ideally, when the danger is over you relax and the excess cortisol signals the hypothalamus to stop the HPA hormone cascade. Many of us get caught in that heightened stress state, never releasing it from our system and returning to neutral. If we don't discharge this energy, the primitive brain locks the experience in our system, allowing the emotions we experienced at the time to remain alive inside of us. Unfortunately, our systems cannot determine the difference between stress due to an actual threat and those stemming from unresolved emotional conflicts or unprocessed trauma. When we hold unresolved emotions in our bodies, we become suspended in a state of overdrive, and many of us stay there in an effort to avoid feeling All The Things. While our body has the incredible ability to both protect *and* heal itself, it can't do both at the same time. When we allow ourselves to experience our full range of emotions, we begin the healing process. This is an awesome start! When we allow ourselves to experience pleasure, it's a game changer.

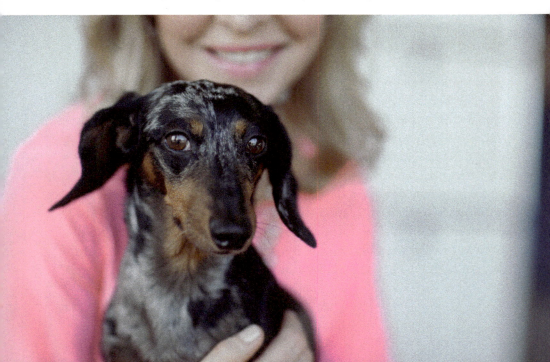

# Shake That Shit Off
# (Or, What My Dog Already Knows)

Hans Selye coined the word "stress" in the 1930s when his research with rats showed that threatening conditions cause hormone secretions that damage organ tissue. Stress has no translation in any other language, the closest being a Chinese word written with two characters, one representing "danger" and the other "opportunity," to signify crisis. I like to think of this as a reminder that stress can be an opportunity. Purging the survival chemicals after a stressful experience sends a message to our primitive brain that we are now safe (phew!). When this happens, our cognitive brain gets the signal to go ahead and process the information and release any associations related to it that are no longer needed. When this happens, the energy of the stressful event is discharged and it can actually lead to feelings of empowerment. In this case, stress can be seen as a healthy way to build feelings of self-confidence (I've got this!).

While our bodies naturally know how to purge survival chemicals after a stressful event, many of us aren't comfortable with what this natural process looks like—your teeth chatter, your knees knock, your hands shake. You may have been taught that shaking is a sign of weakness and you suppress it, but shaking is actually a sign that your body is releasing energy. It's what happens when your fight-or-flight response winds down and you want (and need) for this to happen! I find it super helpful to actually exaggerate whatever is naturally happening in my body to help those stress chemicals sort themselves out.

When an animal experiences a stressful event, it shakes, trembles, runs, or performs some other physical activity to discharge the effect of stress chemicals in its body. It rebalances itself and gets back to the business of being an animal. I recognize this behavior in my dog Gello (pronounced "Jello") all the time. Gello would be super happy to pal about with me everywhere I go, and while we're mostly inseparable, there are occasions I go places where he's not invited. Before I leave, I make a comfy nest for him inside his crate with blankets and a few (or ten) stuffed buddies. I throw in some treats and words of encouragement (for me), because I know that Gello is about to be stressed out of his little doggy mind (think chewed blankets and puddles of slobber). When I come back from my dog-free adventure and unlock his crate, Gello does what we've come to refer to as his "crazy dance." He runs back and forth between his crate and the living room across the house, "rescuing" all his buddies one by one. Gello just celebrated his 13th birthday, so I've witnessed the ritual countless times over the years, but I've gone from thinking "oh fuck, my dog is really crazy" to "wow, my dog is a master releaser." Let's all be Gello!

## Don't Believe Everything You Think

> "… We must challenge our self-defeating behaviors and find new ways of reacting to the everyday events that shape our experience. We must first digest and embrace all the limiting beliefs we've collected throughout the years, and then, ultimately, summon the courage to let go of them all—everything that is covering our true masterpiece."
> — Debbie Ford, *The Best Year of Your Life*

Our beliefs about who we are and what we deserve to experience can be stumbling blocks to truly experiencing pleasure. A belief is a thought we have over and over again, while *limiting beliefs* are misleading conclusions we make about ourselves based on our experiences. We begin collecting these beliefs during childhood and can build pretty impressive collections as we continue to have life experiences. If you are a woman living in our society, you no doubt have had limitless opportunities to build your own collection. It can be hard to recognize our own limiting beliefs because they just seem like the truth to us. These beliefs hide out behind our good intentions that don't manifest. They live within the deeply carved grooves in our brain circuitry, fed by our fear-based thoughts about who we are.

Body shame is a limiting belief woven into the fabric of our culture, and often starts within our own families. I come from a long line of women with a deep sense of body shame, and chances are you do too. The day I overheard our family doctor tell my Grandma Kay, "Heather isn't just chubby anymore, she's fat," wasn't my first experience of feeling shame about my body, but it serves as a good example of how easy it can be to add to your personal collection of limiting beliefs. Ten years of life had taught me that hushed tones rarely meant anything good. So if what Dr. Greene was saying about my body had to be *whispered*, it was really bad. It made me feel ashamed and reinforced the misleading conclusion I had already developed: that my body *itself* was shameful. The fact that I wasn't actually fat (I was a normal kid about to experience a growth spurt) mattered much less to me than how the words made me feel about my body. And that's the thing about limiting beliefs—they *are* real. They are real in that they come with a real and painful experience of fear or hurt or shame in our bodies. But are they *true*?

I carried my limiting belief about my shameful body into my teenage years when a comment from my boyfriend Sven both reinforced this established belief and added to my collection. It was summer and I was sunbathing in Mama Ruth's garden, enjoying the simple pleasures of watching birds fly overhead and feeling the warmth of the sun on my bare skin. I was happy, carefree, and thirsty. As I made my way into the kitchen for a glass of water, I was greeted by the words, "You would be such a knockout if you just lost five pounds." I stood there in my bikini as the hot rush of shame made its way through every inch of my imperfect body. I felt naked, vulnerable, and ashamed. I had allowed myself the pleasure of enjoying my body and feeling comfortable in my own skin, only to be reminded that I was flawed, I was human, I could stand to lose five pounds.

The limiting belief I collected that summer was that I didn't *deserve* to feel pleasure, and for far too many years, I allowed this belief to be true for me. Not only did I decline any and all invitations to summer pool parties throughout my teenage years, I also rarely allowed myself the simple pleasure of feeling the warmth of the sun on my bare skin. My body was something to keep hidden, covered in pants and shirts long enough to hide the arms and legs that would reveal my imperfections to the world, leaving me as vulnerable as I felt standing in my kitchen on that summer day. I remained comforted by the promise of *next* summer being different. I would lose those five pounds and the truths they held about my worth. Next summer would be different, and so would I. The truth about that long-awaited summer? It took decades to arrive and it had nothing to do with those five pounds.

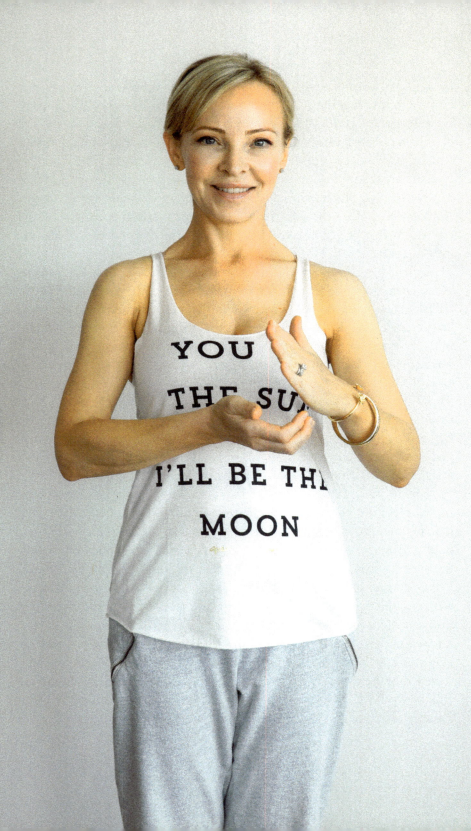

Ready to tackle *your* limiting beliefs so you can get down to the business of honoring your pleasure? You're in luck, because EFT Tapping is an *amazing* way to do that and I'm about to show you how. When we "tap" while focusing on a belief we wish to change, its emotional stronghold weakens. By targeting the emotions and the stress response our beliefs create, the stress response is lowered (or gone altogether) and the limiting belief no longer feels true. You can then create a new, positive belief that *does* feel true. Imagine how much better that would be!

*"Our unprocessed emotions, beliefs, and traumas are still operating and controlling our lives. We need to address them—to look at them, admit they are there, and work through them—in order to clear them."*
— Nick Ortner, *The Tapping Solution*

## Emotional Freedom Technique (EFT) Tapping

I like to think of Tapping as sort of energy medicine meets positive affirmations. Technically, working with psychological issues by Tapping on the meridian acupoints is part of an emerging field known as "energy psychology." Tapping is my go-to method for healing basically anything that might want healing (a headache, a personal relationship, a limiting belief) … but it wasn't always that way. In the beginning I was actually resistant to the whole tapping thing, but it just kept showing up in my life, trying with all its might to get my attention. I gave in (a little) and bought Nick Ortner's *Tapping Solution* book. I let it gather some dust, but I did read it. Cover to cover I read it, and I *loved* it. Still, I didn't tap. I read testimonials and was blown away by the (sometimes miraculous) changes that all kinds of people were making in their lives. Still, I didn't tap. Eventually I did become curious about my behavior, because that's just what I do. My "secret knowing" was telling me that Tapping was something I wanted (and possibly needed). I'm all about collecting new tools for my "wellness toolbox," so why wasn't I *actually* Tapping?

I decided to Google "resistance to tapping" and sure enough it's a thing. Remember in the last chapter when I suggested that becoming curious about how something you might consider "negative" is actually working *for* you? Well, becoming curious about my refusal to tap allowed me to do just that—explore how something in my life was serving me so well, I didn't want to let it go. While I'd been planning to explore Tapping for a variety of issues, there was one thing in particular I wanted to tap on first, and that was my fear of driving. I'd completed the required Driver Ed in high school and drove a bit in my teenage years, but those days were decades behind me. I hadn't actually driven a day of my adult life. City living made it pretty easy to avoid driving altogether, but my husband and I had just bought a house in the Napa Valley. My new life required a car—one that I would have to drive. I'd talked about getting my license for years and even hired a professional driving instructor, but every time that first lesson got close, I rescheduled it. Finally, as our moving date loomed near, I tapped. But, I didn't tap on driving, not at first. I tapped on my *resistance* to Tapping, and that's when things got interesting.

> *There is a pain—so utter—*
> *it swallows substance up—*
> *Then covers the Abyss with Trance—*
> *So memory can step*
> *Around—across—upon it*
> *As One within a Swoon—*
> *Goes safely—where an open eye—*
> *Would drop Him—Bone by bone*
> — Emily Dickinson

As I Tapped through my resistance to Tapping itself, I got super clear on why I wasn't using this technique to get myself into the driver's seat. And, it wasn't what I thought. While I had some legitimate concerns about being on the road (some drivers are assholes, some of them text while being assholes), my driving anxiety was actually based on a fear I held about *myself*. Tapping on my resistance to Tapping allowed me to discover that my unwillingness to drive was less about the actual driving part than it was about keeping myself (and others) safe.

Like many people who have experienced trauma in their lives, I have a history of dissociation—or as I like to think of it, "going to a special place in my head." Our brain's ability to dissociate is actually a vital part of our ingrained survival system, and we all do it from time to time. During a traumatic event, it can help us tolerate what might otherwise be too difficult to bear. Dissociation exists on a spectrum that at one end is quite common (think daydreaming), but on the other end can interfere with day-to-day functioning. I became aware of my own tendency to dissociate while working with a therapist, but it hadn't occurred to me that my fear of driving wasn't based on driving *itself*; rather, it was my fear that I would dissociate while driving (as bad as texting!).

While it was true that dissociation was a coping mechanism I'd relied on at different points in my life, it was *also* true that I already had (and used) lots of tools to support me in remaining present in my body, and in my life. Encouraged by the revelation of what was *truly* holding me back, I was excited to find out what else Tapping could do! I started by Tapping on my belief that I would dissociate while driving. Once this belief no longer felt true, I was able to tap my way into a belief that *did* feel true: that I was calm, present, and confident while driving. I was amazed at how quickly the process actually worked; it took *way* longer to get me to tap in the first place! After one session of Tapping on my resistance to Tapping, followed by two sessions that focused on my fear of dissociating while driving, I was able to book (and keep) my first official driving lesson *and* ace my driving test! What might happen if *you* tapped?

## Your Brain on Tapping

The limbic system or "midbrain" is located between the frontal lobes (the cortex) and the hindbrain (our reptilian brain). This system is the source of our emotions, long-term memory, and is where our negative experiences are encoded. The amygdala is part of the limbic system and it's what signals the brain to mobilize the body in the fight-or-flight response. The hippocampus is also part of the limbic system, and its job is to compare past threats with present signals and to let the amygdala know whether or not the present signal is an *actual* threat. This response evolved to keep our ancient ancestors safe in the face of very real threats to survival (think saber-toothed tigers), but today this response is more likely to be triggered by the overwhelm of our daily lives, as well as our thoughts and limiting beliefs. When we experience a negative emotional state like anger or fear, our brains go on alert, preparing our bodies to fight or flee. The stress response only cares about protecting you, not distinguishing between an actual threat and a perceived threat. Regardless of whether a tiger is indeed chasing you or you are experiencing emotional pain, your stress response is the same—your adrenaline and cortisol rise, your muscles tense, and your blood pressure increases. What that feels like in your body is stress and the ability to take action (fight or flee). Even if it's a lower grade response than being chased by a tiger, the cumulative effect of this constant assault takes its toll on our physical and emotional well-being.

## Like Riding a Bike

The knowledge of how to ride a bicycle is stored in what's called "procedural memory"—a type of implicit (or unconscious) and long-term memory that helps us perform particular types of tasks without conscious awareness of previous experiences. Procedural memory kicks in when the brain needs to keep something current for you. It's super helpful when riding a bike, but kinda tricky when it comes to emotional trauma. When we experience a traumatic event and fight-or-flight isn't an option, we go into the freeze response. When this happens, those memories (big or small) are stored away as procedural memory. The trauma is kept current for you because it was deemed "very important." When this happens, it's as if the experience never really stopped happening for you. That's why when we think of a past trauma, we can so easily relive that same feeling.

Tapping allows us to relocate specific memories out of procedural memory so that they aren't a current event for us any longer. Let that sink in for a moment. It's actually pretty huge, right? When we tap on the acupuncture points, it triggers energy and blood flow throughout the meridians and this tells the amygdala to calm down. When the amygdala gets the message that it's safe to relax, stress is immediately reduced. Tapping as you *intentionally* trigger the fight-or-flight response sends the message that the amygdala can deactivate and with repetition, the hippocampus gets the message that the "danger" is no longer a threat. When we tap the acupuncture points while holding the trauma in mind, we are stimulating the meridian system to restore energetic balance *and* we are reprogramming the brain and body to both act and react differently. This is healing in action!

## Tapping Your Truth

*"The truth will set you free, but first it will piss you off."*
— Gloria Steinem

As you begin Tapping, you might wonder why we are focusing on negative thoughts. I was curious about that too. What about the power of positive thinking or the law of attraction? While our culture emphasizes keeping things positive, the reality is that these "negative" thoughts exist, whether we choose to look at them or not. Positive thinking certainly has its place, but when we get there too quickly after a traumatic event, we risk interrupting the natural process of healing. Instead of thinking about these emotions as either negative or positive, try thinking about them as "the truth." I love what Nick Ortner says about this: "you explore the truth to see how you can change it to a more *empowering* truth." This has been my personal experience of Tapping, and I believe it can be *yours* too. Consider this your safe place to unpack your truths. When it's time to go positive, you'll naturally shift to that perspective.

## 8 Steps + 8 Points: Tapping Quick Start

The EFT Tapping Sequence is designed to hit all the major meridian endpoints, regardless of the issue, making it a super simple process to learn. By the time you read the 8 steps below and follow me through each of the 8 points, you'll have everything you need to start Tapping. Since you go through the same steps for *anything* you want to tap on, you'll get the hang of it pretty quickly. I'm going to walk you through the steps below and then you'll have an opportunity to try it out for yourself!

**Step 1:** Identify your "Tapping Target" and create a reminder phrase. A Tapping Target is the issue you want to tap on and can be absolutely anything (body image, stress at work, food allergies). Not sure where to start? In *The Tapping Solution*, Nick suggests starting with your "Most Pressing Issue," and it always works for me! Just ask yourself the question, "What's bothering me *most* right now?" and start there. Once you've got your Tapping Target, you want to create a "reminder phrase," and this is just a short version of the issue to keep it front and center in your mind. For example, if you have chosen to tap on feeling shame about your body, a reminder phrase might be "this shame I'm feeling" or simply "this shame."

**Step 2:** Once you've identified your Tapping Target and created a reminder phrase, you will rate the intensity of your target on a 0 to 10 Subjective Units of Distress Scale (SUDS). What level of stress does this issue currently generate in you? A 10 would be the most distress you can imagine, and a 0 would mean you don't feel any distress at all. What I love about this part is that sometimes when we begin experiencing relief through Tapping, we forget how intense the issue previously was. As the rating decreases, you have the opportunity to appreciate your progress!

**Step 3:** Once you've identified your SUDS level, the next step is to create a setup statement. Your setup statement should acknowledge the issue you want to address, and be followed by an unconditional affirmation of yourself as a person. Here is an example of a setup statement and affirmation for Tapping on body shame: "Even though I feel shame about how my body looks, I deeply and completely love and accept myself." This part might feel awkward at first, but that's okay! Once you begin to actually *believe* your affirmation, it's going to feel amazing.

**Step 4:** To perform the Tapping setup, use four fingers on one hand to tap the Karate Chop point with the other hand (see image below). The Karate Chop point is on the outer edge of the hand, on the opposite side from the thumb. The same meridians run down both sides of the body, so you can tap on whichever side of the body feels best to you. Repeat your setup statement and affirmation three times aloud, while simultaneously Tapping the Karate Chop point.

**Step 5:** After Tapping on the Karate Chop point and repeating your setup statement and affirmation three times, it's time to start your Tapping rounds. You will move through the eight points of the Tapping sequence (see images below) using your reminder phrase. Your fingertips have a number of energy meridians, so we tap using our fingertips. Some people tap using their index and middle fingers, others tap using all their fingers. It makes no difference at all, so do what feels right for you. Tap 5–7 times each on the meridian points in the following sequence:

- Start of the eyebrow, near the bridge of your nose
- Side of the eye, near your temple

- Under the eye
- Under the nose
- The crease between the chin and lip
- The collarbone
- Underneath the arm
- Top of head

Now, tap 5–7 times on each of the Tapping points on either side of the body (or both) as you work through the sequence. You want to spend enough time Tapping at each point to speak your reminder phrase and really let it sink in, so if it feels right to tap longer, do it!

**Step 6:** Once you've completed two full rounds of Tapping, it's time to notice what's happening for you in your body. Take a deep breath to become fully present and consider whether the issue has shifted.

**Step 7:** How do you feel on the SUDS now? If your number has gone down dramatically, your Tapping has done its job (this sometimes happens quite quickly). If you are only feeling partial relief, continue Tapping a few more rounds. When you feel ready, we will be moving on to positive affirmations.

**Step 8:** I'm a huge fan of this step! Shifting to positive affirmations is an awesome way to close out your Tapping session because it allows you to get in touch with how you actually *want* to feel; that said, it's important not to rush this step. If you begin your positive round and the words aren't ringing true for you, that's a good indication that you probably need to go back to the negative beliefs until they clear.

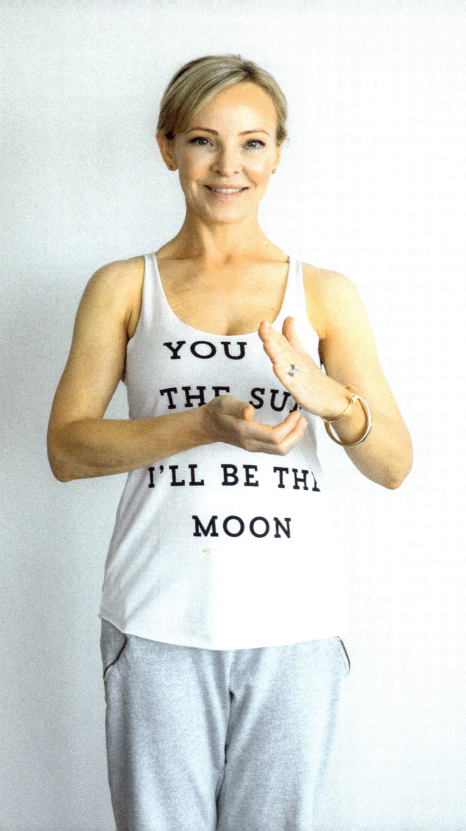

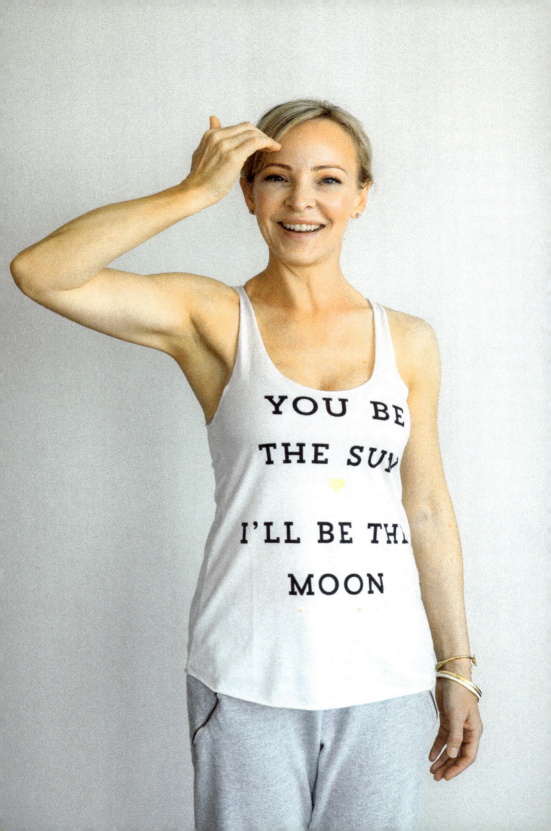

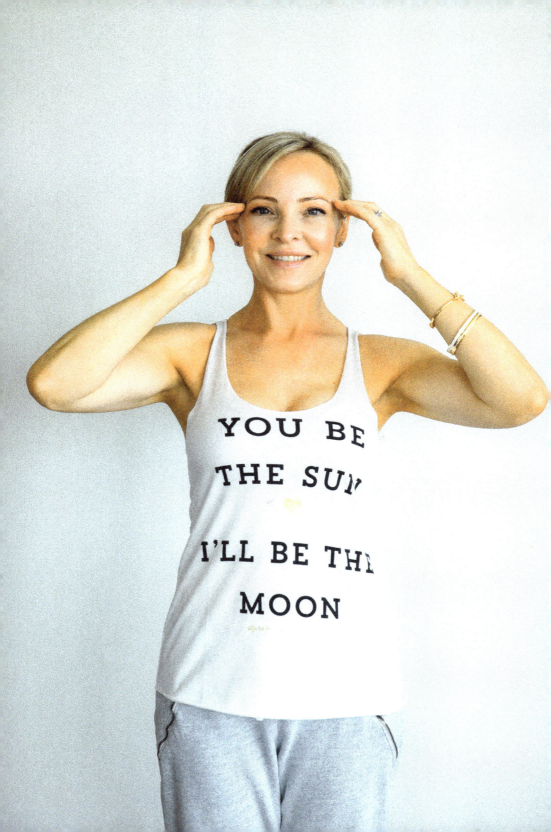

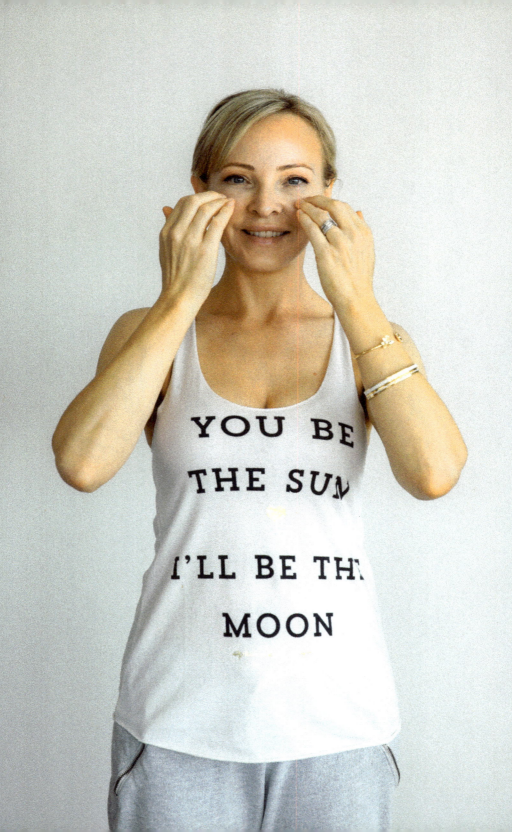

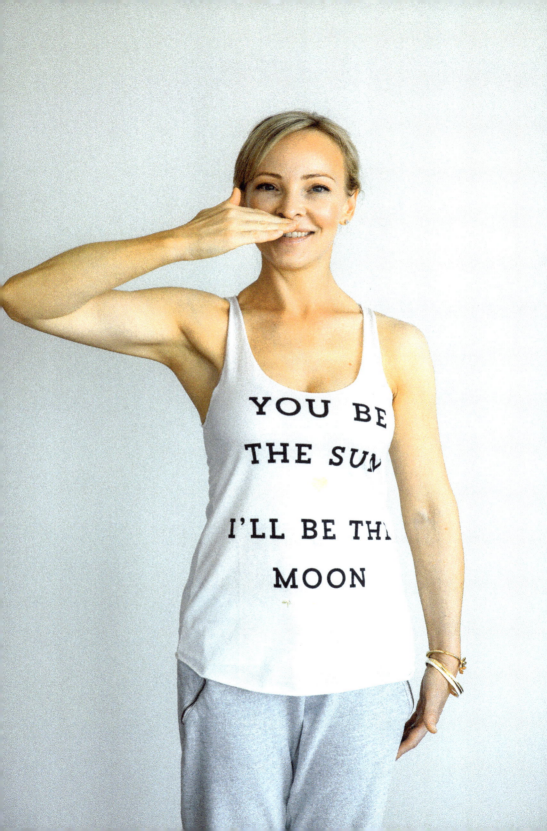

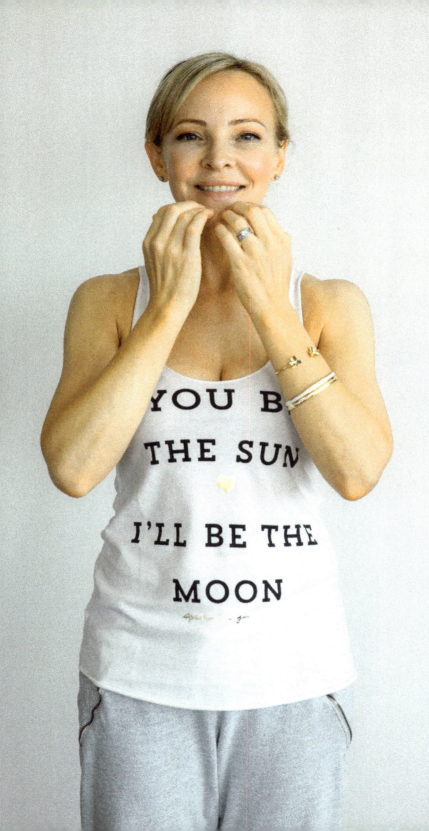

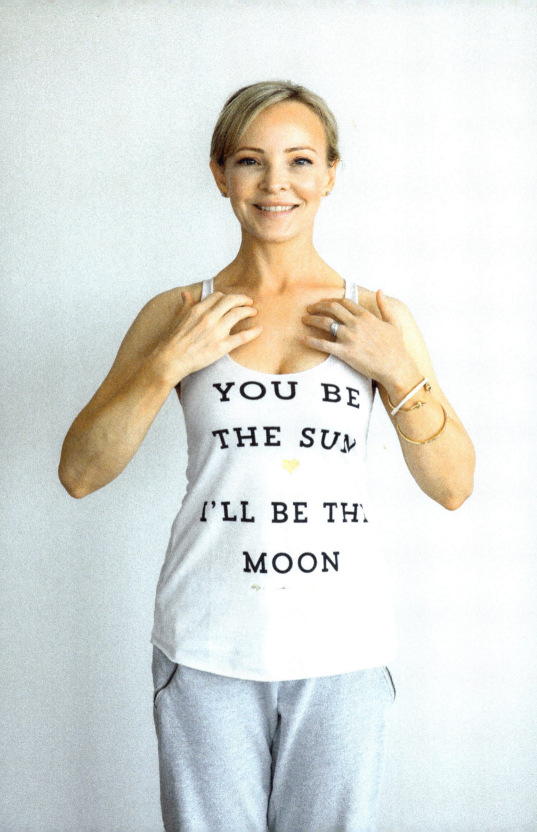

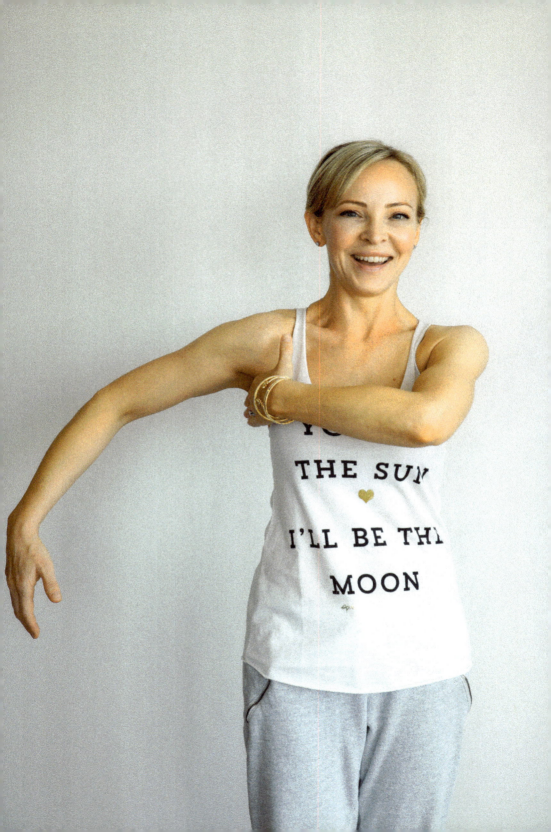

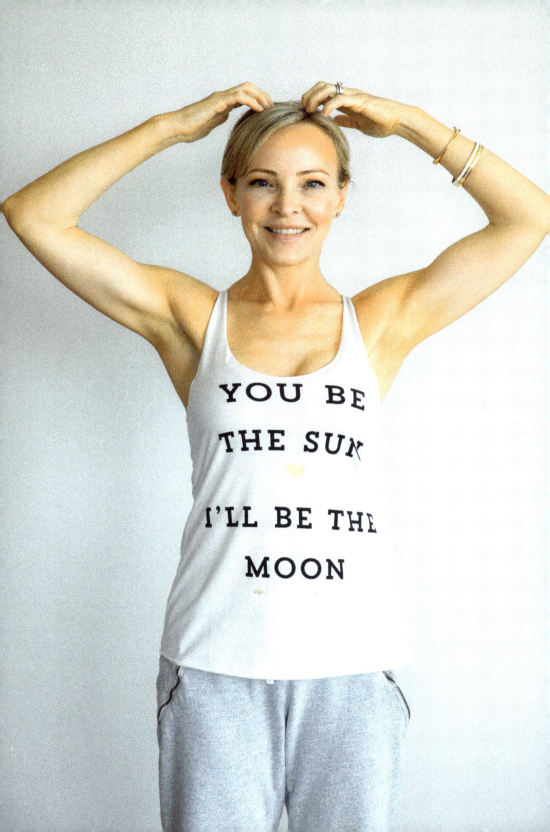

# Tapping Target: Your Limiting Belief

Now that you have a general sense of what the Tapping rounds look like, it's time to tap! Our focus for this first Tapping round is going to be any limiting belief that may be keeping you from experiencing pleasure in your life. While you may have more than *one* limiting belief, go ahead and pick something you'd like to focus on. To illustrate, I'll use my old limiting belief that I don't deserve to feel pleasure. If you happen to have the same limiting belief, go ahead and just follow along. Otherwise, you'll be creating your own setup statement and reminder phrase as we do the following:

**Step 1:** Identify your "Tapping Target." *My Tapping Target is my limiting belief that I don't deserve to feel pleasure.*

**Step 2:** Rate the intensity of your target using the SUDS method.

**Step 3:** Create a setup statement and reminder phrase. *My setup statement is "even though I feel like I don't deserve pleasure, I deeply and completely love and accept myself" and my reminder phrase is "I don't deserve pleasure."*

**Step 4:** Repeat your setup statement three times aloud, while simultaneously Tapping the Karate Chop point.

**Step 5:** Take a nice deep inhale and a long exhale. Begin your Tapping sequence using your reminder phrase.

- Start of the eyebrow, near the bridge of your nose: *"I don't deserve pleasure."*
- Side of the eye, near your temple: *"I don't deserve pleasure."*
- Under the eye: *"I don't deserve pleasure."*
- Under the nose: *"I don't deserve pleasure."*
- The crease between the chin and lip: *"I don't deserve pleasure."*

- The collarbone: *"I don't deserve pleasure."*
- Underneath the arm: *"I don't deserve pleasure."*
- Top of head: *"I don't deserve pleasure."*

Tap 5–7 times on each of the Tapping points on either side of the body (or both) as you work through the sequence. Remember, you want to spend enough time Tapping at each point to speak your reminder phrase and really let it sink in.

**Step 6:** Once you've completed two full rounds of Tapping, it's time to notice what's happening for you in your body. Take a deep breath to become fully present and consider whether the issue has shifted.

**Step 7:** How do you feel on the SUDS now? If your number has gone down dramatically, your Tapping has done its job. If you are only feeling partial relief, continue Tapping a few more rounds. When you feel ready, we will be moving on to positive affirmations.

**Step 8:** You've shifted your issue (congratulations!), now it's time to get in touch with how you *want* to feel. If the positive affirmations feel awkward at first, you might just need a little practice saying nice things about yourself out loud, so give it a round and see what happens. If you flat out aren't buying a word of it, go back a step and tap it out. There is no need to go back and perform a new setup statement as you switch your language to the positive, as it's all part of the same Tapping round. *My positive round goes like this: "I am worthy of pleasure."*

- Start of the eyebrow, near the bridge of your nose: *"I am worthy of pleasure."*
- Side of the eye, near your temple: *"I am worthy of pleasure."*

- Under the eye: *"I am worthy of pleasure."*
- Under the nose: *"I am worthy of pleasure."*
- The crease between the chin and lip: *"I am worthy of pleasure."*
- The collarbone: *"I am worthy of pleasure."*
- Underneath the arm: *"I am worthy of pleasure."*
- Top of head: *"I am worthy of pleasure."*

This first Tapping exercise can be considered a "general" Tapping sequence. It's everything you need to start Tapping and begin to experience relief for a variety of issues. Tapping on a general issue is going to reduce your stress and make you feel better. Once you get used to Tapping, you can loosen it up and expand a bit. Digging deeper into the nitty-gritty details of specific issues is where the gold is. Using the same Tapping Target, here's an example of what an expanded Tapping sequence might look like:

> *My setup statement remains "even though I feel like I don't deserve pleasure, I deeply and completely love and accept myself" and my reminder phrase is "I don't deserve pleasure."*

- Start of the eyebrow, near the bridge of your nose: *"I don't deserve pleasure."*
- Side of the eye, near your temple: *"When I lose those five pounds I'll deserve to feel pleasure."*
- Under the eye: *"I don't deserve pleasure."*
- Under the nose: *"Pleasure makes me feel vulnerable."*
- The crease between the chin and lip: *"I don't deserve pleasure."*
- The collarbone: *"It isn't safe to feel pleasure."*
- Underneath the arm: *"I don't deserve pleasure."*
- Top of head: *"Pleasure makes me feel ashamed."*

### Switching to the Positive

- Start of the eyebrow, near the bridge of your nose: *"I choose to allow pleasure."*
- Side of the eye, near your temple: *"My heart knows I am worthy of pleasure."*
- Under the eye: *"I choose to allow pleasure."*
- Under the nose: *"Pleasure makes me feel safe."*
- The crease between the chin and lip: *"I choose to allow pleasure."*
- The collarbone: *"I deserve to experience all kinds of pleasure."*
- Underneath the arm: *"I choose to allow pleasure."*
- Top of head: *"I am pleasure."*

## Peeling the Onion

As you begin your own Tapping journey, you might notice that sometimes you begin Tapping with one target in mind and then as you tap through the issue, it reveals more layers. You can think of this as "peeling the onion" (onions have *lots* of layers and they sometimes make you cry). Our emotional, physical, and spiritual experiences are often complex, and the feelings that come up for you while Tapping tell a larger story. An example of this is my expanded Tapping sequence above. While the Tapping Target was my limiting belief that I don't deserve to feel pleasure, as I tapped through the rounds, allowing myself to speak the feelings that were coming up for me, my words reveal that I have associated pleasure with feeling vulnerable, unsafe, and ashamed. Why would I welcome pleasure into my life if I were also welcoming *those* feelings? Feelings of being vulnerable, unsafe, and ashamed settled into my body at a very tender age, leaving me highly suspect of anything that might tempt them out of hiding. That pleasure was not welcome to my party seemed a very reasonable decision, but I had it entirely, achingly wrong. Pleasure didn't invite those feelings, it simply shined a light on what was already present inside of me. I like to think pleasure did this so that I would have the opportunity to tap those feelings right on out of there! And so I did. And *you* can too.

## Additional Tapping Resources

If you are working with Tapping on your own, there are all sorts of resources available for you to learn more about it. You can grab a copy of Nick Ortner's book *The Tapping Solution*, or his sister Jessica Ortner's *The Tapping Solution for Weight Loss & Body Confidence* (it's fantastic). You can also find free video tutorials and all kinds of scripts you can tap along with on YouTube. If you are interested in working one-on-one with an EFT professional, you can find certified practitioners at www.eftuniverse.com/certied-eft-practioners.

> "Normally, when we hear the word "pleasure," we think about sex, but sexual pleasure is a whole-body experience of all the senses. All pleasure is sensual in nature as we allow our bodies to dance with the creative energy of the universe."
>
> — Dr. Christiane Northrup, *Goddesses Never Age*

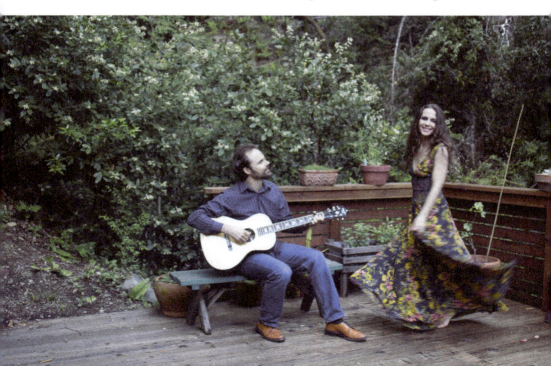

## The Pleasure List

Creating a "pleasure list" is an awesome way to connect with the things in life that bring you pleasure. Shifting your focus, even for a moment, to something you enjoy sends a message to your brain that says "I deserve happiness." And guess what? You do! In no particular order (except coffee), here are ten of my favorite ways to incorporate pleasure into my life that actually have *nothing* to do with having an orgasm:

1. Bulletproof coffee to start my day
2. Morning snuggles with my husband and Gello
3. Walking barefoot: in the grass, on the beach, a country road … anywhere I can!
4. Hugging trees
5. Writing in my gratitude journal
6. Talking with Mama Ruth: by text, by phone, in person … it's all good!
7. Adventuring with Gello
8. My "pleasurable self-care routine" (more about *that* in the next chapter!)
9. Harvesting lemons from my lemon tree
10. Wearing a super cute outfit

## What Brings *You* Pleasure?

Okay, it's your turn! If you have trouble getting started, try making a list of the people (and pets!) who make your heart all warm and fuzzy when you think of them. Then make a list of the places that bring a smile to your face. Keep your list handy so you have access to pleasure any time you need it (a note on your smartphone is perfect). The next time you need to hear the message that you deserve pleasure, grab your Pleasure List and either a) *actually* do something on the list, or b) *imagine* yourself doing something on the list. Turns out you benefit either way! How cool is that?

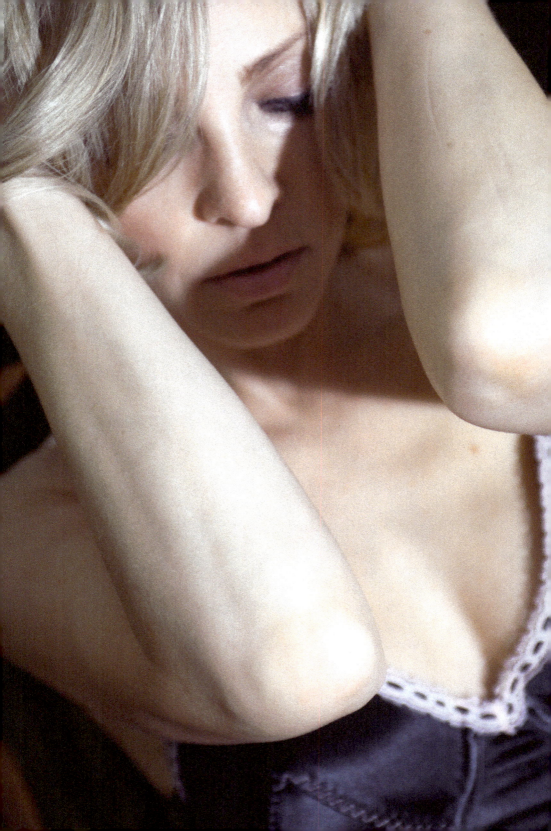

*"The orientation to pleasure is a feminine instinct, and each glorious inch of your body is yours to use for your fulfillment. Women have a greater affinity for pleasure—a drive, an innate understanding of pleasure—simply because they're women. After all, they have an organ on their body whose sole function is pleasure."*

— Regena Thomashauer, *Mama Gena's School of Womanly Arts*

## Finally, the Orgasm Part!

From an Eastern perspective, sexual energy is the same as life-force energy and is one of the most powerful energies we have for creating vibrant health and radiant beauty. Healthy sexual energy allows us to fully experience all the pleasure that is our birthright. When we work with this energy in a conscious way, not only do we open ourselves up to experiencing limitless amounts of sexual pleasure, we also feel more creative, confident, and motivated. You can take those feelings anywhere you want ... imagine the possibilities!

While I'm excited to share my personal experience of working with this vital energy, I find it impossible to talk about sexual pleasure without also bringing attention to just how many of us have experienced sexual trauma in our lives. Statistics from the National Sexual Violence Resource Center state what too many of us personally know to be true:

- That one in four girls will be sexually abused before they turn 18 years old, and that 12.3% of these girls were age 10 or younger at the time of their first rape.
- That more than one-third of women who report being raped before age 18 also experience rape as an adult.
- That health care is 16% higher for women who were sexually abused as children.
- That one in five women will be raped at some point in their lives.
- That in eight out of ten rapes, the victim knew the perpetrator.

# #IAmNotAshamed

> *"Most people don't want to talk about this. Most women are afraid to bring it up, because it can feel too scary and deep. But I know, from personal experience, that this issue is one of the biggest, deepest and most painful obstacles that women face. Not talking about it keeps us in pain."*
>
> — Layla Martin, Creator and Founder of the Tantric Institute of Integrated Sexuality

There is no lucky side when it comes to sexual abuse statistics. If you haven't experienced sexual trauma yourself, you know somebody who has, even if they haven't felt safe enough to tell their story. There are a wide variety of experiences that have the potential to create trauma inside your body. These experiences can range from more obvious traumatic events like rape, incest, and sexual abuse to more subtle forms like being told there is something wrong with your female body, being shamed for your sexuality, and the growing issue of "rape culture" in our society. Healing sexual trauma often requires the support of skilled experts, and while it is beyond the scope of this book to go deeply into such complex territory, I can share with you that I am a survivor of childhood sexual trauma, and the techniques I am presenting here are safe and effective tools that you can use to support the healing process. If you are a woman who has experienced sexual trauma, know that your capacity for healing is limitless!

## My Experience of Healing (Or, The Things I Wish I Knew)

My personal experience of healing sexual trauma gives me the unique opportunity to share what that looked like for me. I was incredibly blessed to have loving, compassionate, and supportive people in my life as I navigated what would be a long and not at all straightforward journey toward healing—a journey I embarked on nearly a decade after the abuse stopped. Unable to speak my story, my story spoke itself. It spoke in my disordered eating. It spoke in my struggles with depression, anxiety, and suicidal ideation. It spoke in my inability to recall small and large details of daily life because sometimes I simply could not stay in my body. I was nineteen and in therapy when I finally felt safe enough to remember, and then share, my story. My story was received under the very best of circumstances, by people who showed up on every level to help me heal, making me not only an ideal candidate for healing, but amongst the lucky few. Even under the very best of circumstances, healing is complicated. Here are some of the things I wish I knew:

> **The effects of sexual trauma show up in weird places:** As I began to make the connection between the sexual trauma I experienced as a young girl and how it was showing up in my life as an adult, I felt overwhelmed, sad, and super pissed off. The symptoms of abuse were showing up *decades* later (sometimes in unexpected ways) and having a significant impact on my present life. Sexual trauma often has psychological, emotional, and physical effects on survivors, and while each of our experiences is unique, there are many symptoms that survivors share. Here's how some of them showed up in my life:
> 
> - **Difficulty concentrating, hyper-vigilance, and an exaggerated startle response:** Going through life this way is tricky and exhausting!
> - **Dissociation:** While helpful during a traumatic event, my tendency to dissociate has affected my intimate relationships, my work, and my ability to recall details of my daily life.
> - **An inability to speak my truth:** When we are silenced by shame it not only hinders our ability to seek the support we need to heal, it can impact our lives on many levels and for years to come. I was not only unable to speak my truth about my abuse, but I found it nearly impossible to speak up in any other capacity in my life.

- **Overwhelming feelings of disgust about my body:** I sought relief from the feelings I had about my body any way I could, but disordered eating, compulsive exercise, and numbing out were my go-to's.

**Healing happens all the time and never.** I am profoundly grateful when I notice healing in my life. This happens all the time because I've taught myself to pay attention. I hardly ever feel disgusted by my body, and when I do I meet that feeling with compassion and melt it away with love. Mindfulness practices allow me to stay in my body so that I can be present for my life and for the people in it. Sometimes I have an effortless ability to speak my truth (which still shocks me). Other times I find it impossible to find the truth within myself, much less say it out loud. When I notice the places that hold the most healing I stay there as long as I can; these moments of noticing are precious and sometimes fleeting. Healing is a practice.

**There are so many ways to approach healing (try them all):** The paths we take on our healing journey will be unique to each of us. From personal experience I believe in trying All The Things, and I've included a list of my favorites for you in chapter seven.

# #MeToo

Billions of people on this planet share the experience of sexual trauma, but our inability to have an open conversation about it is limiting our ability to prevent it, heal it, and integrate it fully into our lives so that we can become whole. Even if we have gotten to a place where it's more common to talk about sexual abuse, there is still shame—a shame we need to heal as a culture for ourselves, our loved ones, and future generations. If you recognize that *you* have a story to tell, please consider this your invitation (your future self is totally rooting for you!).

## Transforming Shame into Love

My hope for all women is that they allow themselves the freedom to experience their own unique beauty, without judgment or shame. Shame thrives in darkness and secrecy. Owning our shame by speaking it out loud can be a powerfully transformative act. In her book *Goddesses Never Age: The Secret Prescription for Radiance, Vitality, and Well-Being*, Dr. Christiane Northrup writes that many women have been shamed by not measuring up to some elusive ideal of beauty, and that unhealed wounds from sexual abuse or shaming can cause a woman to become out of touch with her body. Remember that e-motion (energy in motion) is meant to flow through our bodies. The energy of shame has a particularly tenacious quality to it, but a little gentle coaxing can work wonders. This simple exercise is a really good start.

- Think of something you are ashamed of and go ahead and sit with this feeling of shame for a bit. Breathe into it. Own it.
- See if you can pinpoint where this feeling of shame is hiding out in your body. Can you feel it? Breathe there.
- When you are ready, allow your shame to have a voice: "I am so ashamed of myself for (fill in the blank)." Breathe. Repeat. "I am so ashamed of myself for (fill in the blank)."
- Notice again where this particular feeling of shame makes itself felt in your body. As you feel this shame in your body, breathe into it and whisper the words "I love you right there." Breathe. Repeat. "I love you right there."

# Honoring Your Lady Bits: Grab a Hand Mirror (Yes, Really)

> *"From a mass media saturated with images of what our bodies should look like to our culture's extremely ambivalent attitudes toward sexuality, it is not easy for women to accept, embrace, and enjoy their bodies."*
>
> — Regena Thomashauer (Mama Gena)

I don't recall exactly how I first got my hands on Regena Thomashauer's book *Mama Gena's School of Womanly Arts: Using the Power of Pleasure to Have Your Way with the World*, but I do recall exactly when I slammed that book shut and gave it a good "hell no, I'm not doing that." It was Lesson 4. To be fair, Mama Gena starts the lesson with "this could be a parting of the ways with us ... you can always come back to this one later." We'll see about that, I thought. I shelved this book like I shelved the feelings of shame that the mere *suggestion* of grabbing a hand mirror and looking (like really, really looking) "down there" brought up for me. While I wasn't sure I would ever be up for this crazy little exercise involving a hand mirror and good lighting, there was something Mama Gena said that stuck with me: "And before you bail out of this lesson on me, if you are still with me, let me share one observation that I've noticed since starting my School of Womanly Arts. I have actually found in the last three years of my work, with hundreds of S.G.s (that's "Sister Goddesses" by the way, that's kinda Mama Gena's thing) that the ones who resist this information the most at the beginning actually end up getting the most out of it at the end."

Of course I dusted the book off (eventually) and I did (awkwardly) grab the hand mirror. Now I'm suggesting *you* do the same and here's why: Creating vibrant health and radiant beauty is about a lot of things, but mostly it's about getting to know the one and only *you*. It's about learning to listen to your body's subtle (and not-so-subtle) messages about what it needs and wants to thrive. It's about acknowledging the parts of ourselves that bring us discomfort, so that we can learn to love ourselves anyway. Your lovely lady bits are a part of your body, and if you haven't taken the opportunity to get to know this sacred part of yourself, you may be surprised by what you learn. This, dear one, starts with looking.

## What *Exactly* Am I Looking At?

> *"Self-cultivation is a healthy way to experience sexual pleasure, orgasm, and the release of rejuvenating nitric oxide into the bloodstream ... You are sitting on a throne of gold, the fountain of youth, and it is your erotic anatomy. Explore it and get to know it."*
> — Dr. Christiane Northrup, *Goddesses Never Age*

Despite what the porn industry and their cookie-cutter representations of female sexual anatomy may have led you to believe, the beautiful thing about our lady bits is that everything about them is completely unique to the one and only *you* (this is the part where you pull those panties off and grab your hand mirror):

**Mons Veneris:** Also called the "pubic mound," this is the first thing you will encounter on this intimate journey you are embarking on. In its natural state, your mons veneris will be covered in hair (curly, straight, thick, sparse—it's all good). Pubic hair is nature's way of protecting your sensitive lady bits, and it's also quite sensitive to sensation—something to keep in mind if you are in the habit of grooming this area to within an inch (or less) of its life.

**Labia Majora:** Your labia majora, or "outer lips," will also be covered in pubic hair (or groomed to your preference). Together with the labia minora, they form the labia of the "vulva"—a term that describes the external genitalia of a woman.

**Labia Minora:** When you part the lips of your labia majora, you find your labia minora. Maybe you didn't even have to part your lips to get a glimpse, because besides a huge range of color possibilities (ruby red, pale pink, brown, peach, blue, and more), labia minora come in all kinds of shapes and sizes, all of them uniquely beautiful! You may notice a glossy coating, and this is because your lips are covered with sebaceous oil glands that produce sebum to protect you from infection and disease.

**Clitoris:** At the top of the labia minora is the clitoris, and whether the lovely pearl you see before you is tiny, large, or somewhere in between, she was perfectly designed for one thing and one thing only: *your* pleasure! The 8,000 nerve endings of the clitoris extend down into our bodies hidden from view, but not from sensation. If you picture your clitoris like a wishbone, her "crown" is where the two halves of the wishbone come together, and it is this area that is visible to the naked eye.

**Vagina:** The vaginal opening leads to the vagina—a canal that leads to your cervix. Despite what marketing for "feminine hygiene" products would like you to think, your vagina is the cleanest opening of the body, and your lovely lady bits are entirely self-cleaning.

**Perineum:** The perineum is the skin between your anus and your vagina—a pleasurable spot full of neural activity. In her book *Vagina: A Cultural History*, Naomi Wolf writes that this area is routinely cut during an episiotomy, not just during a difficult childbirth, but often for the economics of hospital time pressures. Many women report diminished sexual sensation after childbirth, especially after undergoing an episiotomy, though they are almost never informed that the procedure will sever a sexual nerve system.

**Anus:** The anus is full of nerve endings that, for some, feel awesome when stimulated. If your favorite spa lists "bunny tail" as part of their waxing services, it's their way of gently letting you know that *everyone* grows pubic hair on their anus. You're welcome.

This exercise can bring up all kinds of feelings for you, every single one of them being absolutely normal. Mama Gena leads a lot of "Sister Goddesses" through this exercise in her *School of Womanly Arts*, and shares these common responses:

- **Yikes!** Okay, breathe. Feeling slightly put off by what your hand mirror reveals is actually a common response (many of us don't look "down there"). Take a scientific approach and just go ahead and observe. Sit in the presence of your own body and see what comes up for you.

- **You are indifferent:** No problem, this is also a common response. Mama Gena believes this reaction is numbness to your own greatness, likely because your potential is so huge (I love that). She recommends the practice of observing other lady bits (paintings and flowers are good places to start) until your approval grows.

- **You feel turned on:** Sweet, you get a gold star! As this process unfolds and you allow yourself to fall more and more in love with this part of yourself, you will become more in tune with yourself and your desires. You may begin to notice a connection between your approval of yourself and your outer experiences in the world as well.

If that exercise was a bit *too* revealing, go ahead and repeat the "Transforming Shame into Love" exercise or do a quick round of Tapping. You can either tap on the specifics of what came up for you as you explored your unique loveliness, or follow along with a more general "I'm uncomfortable" round of Tapping:

*My setup statement is "Even though I'm uncomfortable with how my body looks, I deeply and completely love and accept myself" and my reminder phrase is "I'm uncomfortable with my body."*

As always, begin by repeating your setup statement three times as you tap the Karate Point, then begin your Tapping rounds:

- Start of the eyebrow, near the bridge of your nose: *"I'm uncomfortable with how my body looks."*
- Side of the eye, near your temple: *"I don't think other women look like that."*
- Under the eye: *"I'm uncomfortable with how my body looks."*
- Under the nose: *"I'm not sure I'll ever look down there again."*
- The crease between the chin and lip: *"I'm uncomfortable with how my body looks."*
- The collarbone: *"I'm not sure I'll ever let anybody look down there again."*

- Underneath the arm: *"I'm uncomfortable with how my body looks."*
- Top of head: *"I wish my body looked different."*

### Switching to the Positive

- Start of the eyebrow, near the bridge of your nose: *"Maybe I can look one more time."*
- Side of the eye, near your temple: *"Maybe I was too quick to judge my own body."*
- Under the eye: *"If I look one more time, I might find something about my body that I do like."*
- Under the nose: *"I might not love how my body looks, but I do like the way it makes me feel."*
- The crease between the chin and lip: *"I think I'm going to look one more time."*
- The collarbone: *"I'm going to look for something I love about my body."*
- Underneath the arm: *"I might not love how my body looks, but I love myself anyway."*
- Top of head: *"My body is beautiful because it belongs to me."*

# Crystals + Chakras + Self-Pleasure (Oh My!)

*"The benefits of these exercises are numerous, ranging from the purely physical to the spiritual or energetic ... Using the Jade Egg enables us to access our creative/vital life force consciously and helps us to direct this life force to any part of our body for healing or activation."*

— Saida Desilets, *Emergence of the Sensual Woman*

In chapter three we talked about core strength, personal transformation, and how not to pee your pants. In chapter four we talked about the healing energy of crystals. Now I'm going to introduce you to a (kinda sexy) practice that combines all of those things *and* is believed to increase sexual energy, health, and pleasure.

The use of an oval-shaped stone or "Jade Egg" for improving pelvic health, tone, and suppleness is a Taoist practice that evolved in ancient China. Legend has it that the secret was kept in the Royal Palace and taught only to the queen and concubines of the most powerful nobles. The Jade Egg is made from natural jade (nephrite or jadeite) that is carved into a small egg shape and then drilled from top to bottom, allowing you to thread a string through it. The string helps you to control your experience from practice to removal. On a physical level, the exercises help increase blood and lymph flow through your pelvic floor, increasing vitality and resilience to imbalance. Energetically, jade is considered the health, wealth, and longevity stone. It is traditionally used for increasing courage, wisdom, emotional balance, stamina, and love. In her book *Emergence of the Sensual Woman*, Dr. Desilets writes that the "Jade Egg practice, when done correctly, can be the single most powerful practice to reprogram our beautiful body to know and understand what respectful, loving touch is and a what healthy sexual relationship feels like."

## I Have Reflexology Points *Where?*

Inside the vaginal canal are reflexology points which connect to the heart, lungs, spleen, liver, and kidney. By using the Jade Egg, these points are stimulated, increasing their function in a way similar to acupuncture. The Jade Egg practice keeps our sexual energy circulating throughout our body instead of allowing it to become stagnate or congested in our genitals. Having an awareness of the physical and emotional aspects of each point can help us form a deeper connection with our most intimate anatomy, empowering us to do our own deep healing.

>    **Heart:** Located at the cervix itself. The heart point is associated with the feeling of joy and when balanced, allows us

to feel an abundance of love. When out of balance, you might feel unhappy or restless and experience an irregular heartbeat.

**Lungs:** Located at the top area of the vagina and the area around the cervix. The emotion associated with this point is sadness. When out of balance, you may feel sad or detached and experience a lowered immune system, especially in connection with your respiratory organs. When balanced, you are more at ease with yourself and others.

**Spleen:** Located at the top and third segment of the vagina. The spleen point is associated with overthinking or worry, and when out of balance you may experience digestive issues. When balanced, you feel an inner peace.

**Liver:** Located at the middle and second segment of the vagina (the G-spot area). The liver point is associated with anger and when out of balance, your anger may become explosive or bitter. Balanced, you can express this healthy emotion constructively and (you'll like this one) your skin looks glowy.

**Kidney:** Located at the opening and first segment of the vagina. The kidney point is associated with fear and when out of balance, you may experience trouble with your libido and frequent urinary issues. Balanced, the kidney point nourishes the entire reproduction system.

## *Your* Jade Egg: Purchasing, Preparing, Practicing

As the Jade Egg practice becomes more mainstream, we have an opportunity to explore a lot of different perspectives on the benefits of practice. It's important to educate yourself not only on safe practices, but to decide for yourself if this is the right practice for you at this time. If you have unresolved issues stemming from sexual abuse or trauma, please consider the Jade Egg a complementary tool best used together with the support of a qualified professional to support you on your healing journey. Working with a jade egg is more than just putting a stone in your vagina! There are entire books written about the many benefits and various practices, and while this isn't that book, I find these ones super helpful:

- *The Illustrious Jade Egg: Why Women Rave About It & Everything You Need to Get Started.* This e-book was written by Saida Desilets, PhD, and you can get your hands on your copy by visiting her website, saidadesilets.com. I recommend this book because not only is Dr. Desilets considered the world-leading authority on the practice and offers everything you'll need to get started, but also because I really like her approach. After earnestly following a couple of Taoist books on female sexuality (both written by men) and working with a male teacher whose methods were as confounding as the books, she decided that instead of following the "Ovarian Kung fu" instructions, she would follow her own body's wisdom (I love that). She has been a contributor to Dr. Christiane Northrup's books *The Secret Pleasure of Menopause* and the revised classic *Women's Bodies, Women's Wisdom.* She teaches an adapted version of the ancient Taoist Jade Egg practices she calls "The Desilets Method."
- *The Emergence of the Sensual Woman: Awakening our Erotic Innocence.* Also by Dr. Saida Desilets, this book is a more comprehensive guide with over 60 Jade Egg practices. As awesome as that is, this book is really so much more. In the pages of this book, Dr. Desilets invites us to ignite our own inner wisdom and explore our unique journey of self-discovery and self-cultivation.

You will, of course, want to purchase your Jade Egg from a reputable source (your lovely lady bits will thank you!). One thing to be on the lookout for is that you are purchasing certified pure natural jade (nephrite or jadeite). Less reputable vendors may sell other stones and call them jade, while others even dye their eggs to give them a "jade" color (dying eggs is for Easter, not your vagina!). You also want to make sure that you are purchasing a Jade Egg that has been drilled. You won't always need to use it, but you do want to feel confident about removing your Jade Egg. A drilled egg allows you to use fresh string (essential for hygiene) with each use and comes in handy if you are unable to "lay your egg" with ease. My favorite reputable sources are:

> **Saida Desilets, PhD:** You can purchase a Jade Egg as well as explore some pretty amazing course offerings on Dr. Desilet's website saidadesilets.com.
>
> **Layla Martin:** Layla is the creator and founder of the Tantric Institute of Integrated Sexuality, and you can visit her at layla-martin.com to shop for your Jade Egg *and* get two free instructional videos. If you feel inspired (Layla has that effect), she also teaches a seven-week Jade Egg Masterclass for women (read: she knows her way around a Jade Egg!).

Once you've purchased your Jade Egg, you'll want to clean it properly before your first use. Here's how you do that:

- Place your Jade Egg in a pot of cool tap water, making sure there is about half an inch of water above the egg.
- Bring the water to a boil and let the Jade Egg boil for about 10 minutes.
- Carefully remove the egg with a spoon and let it cool. You *definitely* want your egg to be fully cooled, so please don't skip this part!
- Next you will want to cut either unflavored floss or silk string (the length of your arm is good) and pull it through the drilled hole in your Jade Egg. You will then knot the loose ends, making sure the knotted part is not next to the egg, but at the end of the string.

- Your Jade Egg is now ready to use! Before practicing, please read through this list of precautions: For hygienic purposes, it's not advised to use the Jade Egg while on your period. Please use extra caution if you have an IUD and abstain altogether if you are pregnant.

Be sure to clean your Jade Egg after practice by removing the floss or string and rinsing thoroughly with warm water. Like any energetic stone, your egg also likes the occasional salt bath.

## Practicing Pleasure

*"Let your pleasure be a prayer. Let the mundane become mystical. When it comes to your light, you mustn't tone it down. Burn hotter."*
— LiYana Silver, *Feminine Genius*

Working with the Jade Egg gives you an opportunity to listen to your body, and that actually starts with a "yes" or a "no." I was introduced to this idea through Dr. Desilets' book on the Jade Egg practice, and it's such an amazing way for us to learn (or relearn) that when it comes to our sexuality, our bodies have first say. A simple way to do this is to begin your practice by placing one hand on your heart, your other hand on your vulva, and taking a few long deep breaths as you consider whether or not your body wants to explore this practice. Don't underestimate the power of giving yourself a choice.

**You Will Need:**
- Your Jade Egg
- Unrefined Coconut Oil
- A comfy spot to practice (you'll be lying down)
- An open heart (and mind!)

**How-to:**

- **Warm Your Jade Egg:** You can do this a couple of different ways. I personally like to place my egg on my heart before my practice, but placing your egg in a cup of warm water certainly does the trick.
- **Breathe Your Intention:** Have both your Jade Egg and coconut oil handy, then lie on your back in a comfortable position. Place one hand on your heart and one hand on your vulva. Take several long deep breaths as you set your intention to welcome pleasure.
- **Breathe Your Egg:** When you are ready, gently bring your Jade Egg to the opening of your vagina and begin to gently move your egg in a circle. Take a few more long deep breaths as you continue to circle, and then relax for a moment before you move on to the first pleasure practice.

**Sipping Your Egg**

- **On an Inhale:** Gently squeeze the tip of your Jade Egg with your inner labia. As you exhale, relax your grip and feel your vaginal canal yawn open. On the next inhale, gently squeeze again. Do this for several in- and out-breaths. When you are ready, you can apply light pressure with the hand that is holding the Jade Egg and encourage it to move inwards. Once the egg is in, bring one hand to your heart, one hand to your vulva, and take several long deep breaths.
- *Your* **Pleasure Practice:** What comes next is up to *you.* You can either get up and wear your egg around for a bit, consider your practice complete and move on to "Lay Your Egg," or enjoy a Sacred Yoni Bath.
- **Lay Your Egg:** I find the easiest way to do this is to come into a squatting position and bear down, but I welcome you to find your own best way. Whether you are squatting or lying

down, just gently pull on the string as you push down with your pelvic floor. In time, you will likely be able to "lay your egg" without the extra help of your string.

## Sacred Yoni Bath

*"The flower blooms because she is the perfume she loves."*
— Rumi

*Yoni* is the Sanskrit word for vagina and translates to "sacred gateway to life" (I like that). I think it's lovely to incorporate both rose essential oil and rose petals into my Sacred Yoni Bath, but I'm fancy like that. Go ahead and consider it optional, but amazing. Historically, the rose has served as a symbol of love and inspiration. Rose oil has a restorative and elevating effect on the spirit and emotions, and is also considered an aphrodisiac, which makes it perfect for this (kinda sexy) bath.

In energy medicine, the meridians most involved in sexuality are the kidney, spleen, and liver meridians. The kidney meridian is considered the storage area of our sexual energy; the spleen meridian bolsters the kidney meridian's function; and the liver meridian opens blocked energies while supporting the muscles and ligaments involved in sexual function. During your Sacred Yoni Bath, you will be opening up your sexual energy through use of the Jade Egg and gently massaging your sexual meridian points. You can either enjoy this bath *after* warming up with your Jade Egg (in which case your egg is already inside you), or as a stand-alone practice.

### You will need:

- 1–2 cups Himalayan or Epsom Salts
- 6–8 drops Rose Essential Oil
- Fresh or Dried Rose Petals
- Jade Egg

**How-to:**

Set the mood with soft lighting, candles, and soothing music—your pick! Begin filling your tub with warm water, adding your salts and essential oil, and if you aren't already wearing your Jade Egg from the previous practice, gently place your Jade Egg into the water (a cold jade egg is not ideal!). Once your bath is ready, carefully step into the tub and settle in with several long deep breaths. Once you feel ready, you can perform the same "sipping method" from the previous exercise and you'll be ready for your Sacred Yoni Bath:

- Place your hands open at the insides of your feet. With your hands spread, draw them very slowly and deliberately up the insides of your legs to the tops of your inner thighs.
- Acupressure points for the kidney, spleen, and liver meridians are also located on the creases where your legs and body join. Gently press or massage along the creases to stimulate the energies in these meridians.
- Massaging any tender points on your pelvic bone also keeps the pathways clear so that sexual energies are allowed to flow freely.
- When your Sacred Yoni Bath is complete, you can decide to wear, or lay, your Jade Egg.

## The Jade Egg & Magical Thinking

Whether or not you believe your crystal has magical powers, the practice of tuning into yourself in this intimate way can be profoundly healing. My personal experience of the Jade Egg practice was that I felt empowered to release old traumas and negative sexual associations, ultimately transforming them into positive, life-affirming, pleasurable associations. A Jade Egg practice can be experienced in many ways. I like to think of it as a journey of *you* coming home to yourself. Experiencing sexuality on your own terms while practicing unconditional self-love is one of the potent possibilities of this "magical" practice.

# Follow Your VPA

> *"Our vaginal pulse is our inner barometer and indicator of our life force. It is a felt sense that not only lets us know how safe and valued we are but also connects us to the beauty and joy of living in a body. We can trust this pulse—this life force. You will find that it brings you a great deal of pleasure and delight."*
> — Dr. Christiane Northrup, *Making Life Easy*

Follow my what?! Sex researchers call it the vaginal pulse amplitude (VPA), and they even have a fancy device called a vaginal photoplethysmograph to measure its strength. If you have a vagina, you have a VPA. So, what does it feel like and how exactly do you follow it? Your vital life force is unique to you and you will feel it in *your* very own way. When a woman experiences something pleasing, she can actually experience a distinctive pulse in her vagina. Even if you aren't currently aware of it, once you allow yourself to tune in to it, it will probably feel familiar to you. Pay attention and you'll have no trouble feeling it, and you will begin to notice when you feel the pulse most strongly. The vaginal pulse can be felt when we feel emotionally safe, sexually turned on, and we can also feel it in entirely nonsexual ways.

In her book *Feminine Genius: The Provocative Path to Waking Up and Turning on the Wisdom of Being a Woman*, LiYana Silver refers to it as the "Oracle Between Your Thighs." She writes, "Your own inner knowing can be clarified, catalyzed, and inspired from your trusted sources *out there*, but its source is within you ... your own personal Oracle is within you. It is right where the Divine placed it so reverently and irreverently, right at your South Pole, in every wise cell of your naughty bits." You can start by beginning to notice what turns you on, what makes you feel most alive. If you can begin to pay attention and notice when this happens, you can use it to guide your life. When you feel your own VPA it's an indication that you are headed in the right direction; go toward that!

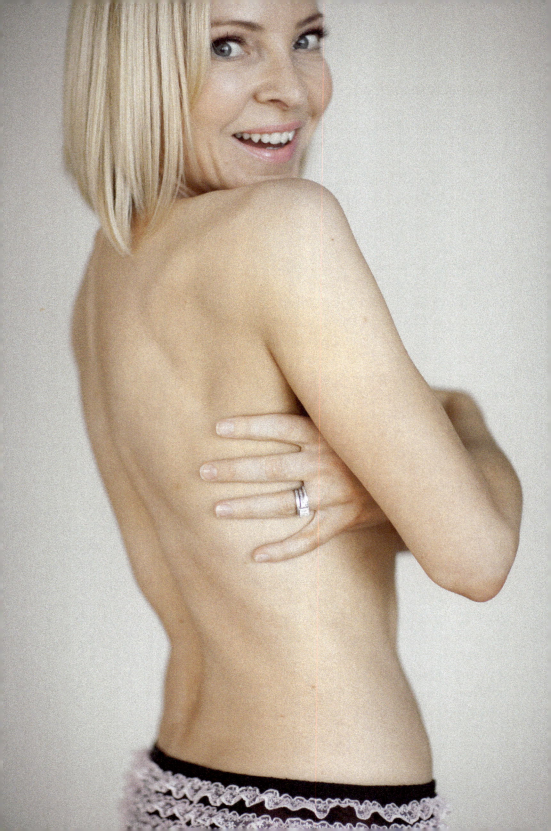

# Chapter Six
# Love Yourself Up: Beauty Rituals from Head to Toe!

**I'm pretty sure** it all started with my Grandma Kay, who, if you came close enough to her velvety soft cheek, emitted the sweetest hint of Oil of Olay—the original pink one. Grandma Kay was my first experience of what I considered a "fancy lady." She had a separate soap just for her face and a Kelly green vanity filled with makeup palettes from Lancôme Paris to "put her face on." I loved watching her perform her beauty rituals, which always started with a splash of Revlon's Jean Naté. There seemed to be no rush, though it didn't take too long (she had a job at NASA to get to after all)—just mindful attention to the details that had a sort of meditative quality to it. I was altogether enchanted and made my mind up early on that I would be a fancy lady too.

In the summertime Grandma Kay would pick a bucket of lemons from her backyard and squeeze them all by hand, then rinse the juice through my long blonde hair to create natural highlights. Afterward, I'd prop myself up on the back of the couch while she brushed out my tangles and gave me what I now know was a proper blowout. What I knew then was that I was loved. In the evenings we would watch old movies and take turns giving manicures, or tickling each other's arms and snuggling. This ritual also included dipping into Grandma Kay's (not-so-secret) stash of fancy chocolates. Thanks to all the happy hormones we generated, I have super positive associations with self-care. I also believe there is magic in the simple act of pampering yourself and the ones you love.

When my Grandma Kay was nearing the end of her long battle with non-Hodgkin's lymphoma, we turned to the rituals we created when I was just a girl. With delicate attention to detail, the act of washing my grandmother's face or tending to her nails became a meditation offering profound comfort. The familiar feeling of her graceful hands drawing themselves up and down my arm was a language we were able to speak when grief took our words.

## A Fancy Lady in a Modern World

*"What I put on my face is as important as what I eat off my plate!"*
— Alexandra Jamieson, author of *Women, Food, and Desire* and creator of Her Rules Radio

In the previous chapter you learned how cultivating pleasure boosts your health and happiness, increasing your levels of nitric

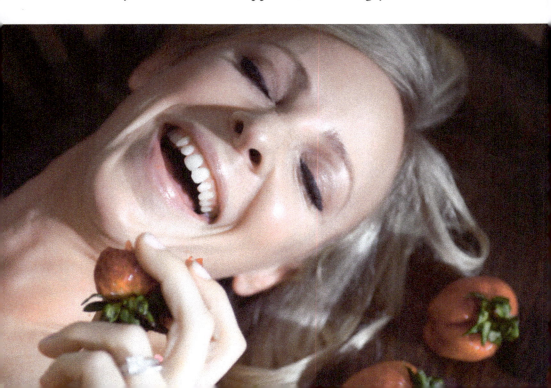

oxide and setting the stage for all manner of awesome things to happen in your body. Pleasure is a vital companion on your personal path to vibrant health and radiant beauty. Taking time to tend to your body is a powerful act of self-love and one of my *very* favorite ways to intentionally bring more pleasure into my own daily life. The best way to enhance our experience of self-care is to remain mindful that our skin absorbs *everything* we put on it. That means that what we put on it matters (a lot).

Losing my beloved Grandma Kay to cancer is one of the things that inspired me to advocate for more awareness around the health and safety of our personal care products and cosmetics. We haven't passed a federal law regulating the beauty industry since 1938. We have introduced over 85,000 chemicals into commerce since World War II, and 80 to 90% of them have never been tested for safety and human health. While the E.U. has banned or regulated more than 1,300 ingredients in personal care products, the U.S. has only banned 11. When you are dealing with chemicals that are carcinogenic, interfere with hormones (endocrine disruptors), or are toxic to your nervous system, the goal is to minimize exposure as much as possible. The beauty industry is essentially unregulated, and this means that cosmetic companies can legally put toxic ingredients into the products we use every day and they don't even have to list them on the label. According to the FDA, "It is the manufacturer's and/or distributer's responsibility to ensure that products are labeled properly." Well, that's not good enough for me, and it's not good enough for *you* either. Lucky for us, these companies agree:

> **Beautycounter:** In addition to creating some of the most luxurious clean beauty products on the market, Beautycounter puts an enormous amount of energy and resources into advocating for legislation and labeling that will help us feel better about the products we put on our bodies. Their banned ingredients list is one of the most thorough in this space, with a "never list" of 1,500 toxic ingredients they refuse to use in their products because they want to keep you safe. It's

awesome when you find a line of products that makes giving up a beloved standby in the name of health easy (no small task). It's also awesome when that same line of products offers clean choices for not just you, but your whole family.

I'm such a fan of Beautycounter that when fellow IIN health coach (and badass wellness warrior) Alexandra Jamieson asked me to join the mission, I partnered with them to personally get safer beauty into the hands of my family, friends, and clients. I can't live without: their face oils, mists, and masks. I keep all three lines on hand (brightening, plumping, and balancing) so I'm covered for any skincare scenario. The Charcoal Cleansing Bar is *everything* (it's Mama Ruth's must-have), and the California girl in me can't resist the Ocean & Pacific makeup palette.

**Living Libations:** I first discovered Living Libations in nutrition school, when "Renegade Beauty" Nadine Artemis was a guest teacher. A renowned holistic health expert and author, Nadine offered a new model for thinking about beauty, health, and body care. I was intrigued, but not yet fully aware of the deep impact her teachings would have on me. She taught that true beauty is not applied, but expressed from within; and that when we are nurtured by nature we allow the life force of flowers, plants, the sun, and water to revive the body and skin. Her words spoke to a part of me that longed to remember the truth of this. The part of me that had turned its back on this wisdom, tempted away by quick-fix promises and cookie-cutter ideals set forth by fashion and beauty magazines. I accepted Nadine's invitation to rediscover (and celebrate) my own unique beauty, to approach my self-care and nourishment in a more holistic way. In that seemingly simple choice, a missing component in my own healing was revealed.

Nadine's concept of eating for beauty informed my own philosophy, inspiring me to nourish myself in an entirely new way. I gained firsthand knowledge of the healing power of self-care and along the way discovered my own unique path to vibrant health and radiant beauty. Consider the wild-crafted and organically grown Living Libations line of products your personal invitation to do the same. I can't live without: her entire line of oral care, body care bundles (especially the Breast Care and Seasonal Beauty kits), the essential oil kits, and her recently released book *Renegade Beauty*.

**Weleda:** Philosopher and scientist Dr. Rudolf Steiner recognized that the human body was a part of nature and that reconnecting with the natural world is the best way to bring our bodies into balance. From the late 1910s, Steiner worked with doctors to create a new approach to medicine, and in 1921, his collaboration with a team of scientists and Dr. Ita Wegman (one of the first women physicians in Europe) brought about the creation of the pharmaceutical company Weleda, which now distributes natural medicine products worldwide. They planted the first biodynamic gardens (which are still cultivated today) and choose handpicked, wild-crafted, biodynamic, or organically grown ingredients for their products whenever possible. They also believe that their intentions infuse their products and allow *your* beauty to shine (naturally, I love that).

Weleda was popular amongst Mama Ruth's hippie friends when I was growing up, and now I understand the fuss. I can't live without Skin Food because it's one of the most versatile products on the planet. I've used it as a facemask, hair helper, lip healer, and cuticle soother. They make a body oil to support pretty much anything you feel needs supporting. My personal favorites are the muscle-soothing Arnica Massage Oil, detoxifying Birch Cellulite Oil (the scrub is amazing too!), heart-opening Wild Rose Body Oil, and regenerating Pomegranate Body Oil.

Throughout this chapter I'll show you how I incorporate my favorite clean beauty products into my self-care routine to nourish my skin from head to toe. Not sure about the safety of a product you want to use? Check the Environmental Working Group's Skin Deep Cosmetics Database at www.ewg.org.

## Love the Skin You're In

*"If you feel some insecurity or dissatisfaction about your skin, know that the cosmetics industry markets to these worries with their skin type hype. Dermatology, the science of skin, has no standard objective measure of "skin type." The skin type classifications (dry, normal, sensitive, combination, oily, and acne-prone) are mere constructs of cosmetics manufacturers. Skin type is a marketing tactic they use to sell products—products that cause the issues they claim to resolve."*
— Nadine Artemis, *Renegade Beauty*

When author and wellness expert Nadine Artemis was a guest teacher at my nutrition school, her lecture on skin health inspired me to not only free my bathroom of toxic beauty products, but to free my mind of outmoded ways of thinking about skin care. She spoke of beautiful skin being the perfect poise of what you put on *it* and what you put in *you*. As you find that balance, your skin becomes strong, resilient, and radiant, because *that* is the true nature of skin. From this perspective, an oily t-zone, and sensitive, dry, or acne prone skin can be looked at as symptoms of imbalance. While these symptoms can be addressed in a number of ways, setting aside toxic skin care in favor of high-quality, clean beauty products and nourishing your body with foods that work best for the one and only you, is the perfect first step. When we create an ideal environment for our cells by providing a good balance of water, oxygen, and nutrients, our bodies thrive and our skin glows. As you explore this chapter, I invite you to set aside your beliefs about your skin and become curious about what your body might be telling *you*.

# Beauty Rituals from Head to Toe: You Glow, Girl!

In my teenage years I devoured fashion magazines, paying particular attention to the beauty tips and step-by-step instructions for the "ultimate DIY facial." I saved up to buy all manner of scrubs, masks, lotions, and potions, and even got mixy in Mama Ruth's kitchen when I'd stumble across a recipe for a homemade version. I delighted in my weekly home facials and the tradition of self care lovingly instilled in me by my Grandma Kay. My friend Susan treated me to my first professional facial at the spa in San Francisco's upscale I. Magnin department store (it was fancy and I was hooked). I love *everything* about a professional facial—the pampering, the promise of renewed beauty, and not least of all the opportunity to get the latest scoop on skincare from the esthetician. I always walk away from my spa experience with some little nugget of inspiration from the professionals who make their living making our skin glow. I love passing on juicy beauty tips, and this pro-style step-by-step at-home facial is full of them (you're welcome).

**The Basics:**

- a heatproof bowl strong enough to withstand boiling water
- bath towel and a washcloth or two
- cotton rounds
- cleanser
- exfoliator
- face oil or balm for the massage part (my favorite!)
- mask
- toner or hydrosol
- serum
- moisturizer

**Extras If You Are Fancy Like That:**

- facial-cleansing brush
- pro-style facial steamer
- flowers, herbs & essential oils for your facial steam
- a gemstone facial roller (trust me, you want this)

While I love a facial with all the bells and whistles, if I'm pressed for time I opt to skip a step or two rather than skipping my pleasurable self-care altogether. This allows me to enjoy the benefits (glowy skin, relaxed vibe) while still tending to the details of my sometimes busy life. If this approach seems more doable to you, check out my "Quick Tips."

**Step 1: Set the Scene**

When you treat yourself to a professional facial, the first thing your aesthetician will do is set the spa scene and tuck you into a cozy blanket cocoon. While a blanket cocoon is impractical and tricky for a home facial, you can still create a spa-like atmosphere by playing your favorite music, lighting a few candles, or diffusing essential oils.

**Step 2: Evaluate Your Skin**

The ancient art of face mapping is a fantastic way to evaluate your skin during your home facial and good practice for taking an outside-in and inside-out approach to beauty. With roots in both Traditional Chinese Medicine and Ayurveda, face mapping is one of the tools practitioners use to evaluate the health of our internal systems. Where we break out, rash, or wrinkle are seen as clues to what our body needs to find more balance.

> **T-Zone:** Consisting of the nose, forehead, and chin, the T-Zone has the highest concentration of oil glands on the face. The forehead relates to our nervous and digestive systems, and frequent breakouts in this area may indicate a need to improve

your pathways of elimination and reduce your stress. Blemishes between your eyebrows or nose area can be associated with an imbalance in the kidney, stomach, or spleen. Consider yoga, meditation, and breath work for reducing stress, and show your organs some love by cutting down on your consumption of alcohol and upping your intake of greens and essential fatty acids.

**Cheeks:** An imbalance in your liver or lungs can show up on your cheeks. Your lungs love deep breathing and fresh air, while your liver appreciates your ability to release unexpressed anger. Spots on your cheeks that show up closer to your nose can be due to an imbalance in the small intestine. Try favoring drinks at room temperature over colder options and see if that works for you. It's also good to keep in mind that dirt from your cell phone or pillowcases can cause blemishes on your cheeks, and that's a really easy fix.

**Jaw Area:** Breakouts below the temple and down to your jaw area can indicate an imbalance in your large intestine or colon. Try adding fermented foods to your already abundant intake of organic vegetables (you *are* doing that, right?) and add a probiotic to your daily supplement regime. Remember, everybody loves to poop.

**Chin:** Linked to the ovaries, breakouts on the chin or along the sides of the chin are common for women struggling with hormonal imbalance. In addition to hormones, blemishes on the jaw line and chin can be caused by candida and yeast overgrowth. Reducing sugar and following an anti-candida diet can be helpful.

## Step 2: Cleansing Ritual

The ritual of cleansing is a fresh start in the morning and a blessing at night. I love the luxurious feel of cleansing oil (simple raw honey is also a favorite), but any gentle wash you prefer is perfect.

Begin washing your face, neck, and décolleté in upward, circular motions. Using a medium pressure will help to stimulate your facial muscles, giving you a lifted and toned appearance. For all the steps that follow, keep in mind that your neck and décolleté love attention too, so don't stop at your face!

**Quick Tip:** You can opt to use a micellar cleansing water with cotton rounds for a quick but thorough cleansing, and then move on to Step 3. Micellar water looks and feels like plain old water, but it's made up of microscopic oil molecules called micelles suspended in soft water that attach to dirt, grime, and makeup, leaving your skin clean and nourished. It's pretty brilliant.

**Pro Tip:** I've been a huge fan (and loyal client) of aesthetician Shelley Costantini for over a decade. A bit of a rock star among Bay Area lovelies who take pride in their "bella pelle" (that's Italian for beautiful skin), Shelley opened her popular BellaPelle Skin Studio in the heart of San Francisco's Union Square in 2002. According to Shelley, performing a double cleansing is ideal for your bella pelle. The second cleanse will "treat" the skin, making it a good time to use a cleanser with either oil-controlling acids, brightening, or moisturizing ingredients depending on your needs. This is also a good time to use your facial cleansing brush (I love my Clarisonic).

## Step 3: Exfoliation

Exfoliation is an awesome way to expose new skin, regenerate skin cells, and enhance the benefits of your lotions and potions. It does this by removing the upper layers of dead skin and speeding up cellular turnover; it also stimulates the production of new collagen fibers. All this is good news for your glowing skin! You can approach exfoliation in one of two ways:

> **Manual:** If you prefer the satisfying feel of a "scrub," you might opt for a physical exfoliator. Keep in mind that if a scrub is too abrasive, it can leave scratches on your skin or even break blood vessels (yikes). Those with sensitive skin sometimes find a facial brush or washcloth does the trick for them.

**Chemical:** A chemical exfoliation goes a bit deeper and utilizes acids derived from fruits, nuts, milks, sugars, or plants. While alpha hydroxyl acids (AHAs) help exfoliate, beta hydroxyl acids (BHAs) such as salicylic acid can help clear out excess dirt, oil, and impurities. Enzymes from fruits such as papaya and pineapple are pretty amazing for super soft, renewed skin.

Both manual and chemical exfoliation are great options, so pick your personal favorite. If you have sensitive skin but love a scrub, try the pro tip(s) below. For a physical exfoliation, take some scrub in your fingertips and wet your hands slightly. Using a gentle touch, move in circular motions around your face (avoid the eye area), neck, and décolleté. Chemical exfoliants should be carefully applied using the product's instructions (leaving it on longer is *not* better). Gently remove with warm water and a washcloth.

**Quick Tip:** If you're pressed for time, try multitasking with an exfoliator that doubles as a mask. When you do this you can either skip the steam in Step 4, or try a quick steam by letting a warm washcloth cool over your face before applying your exfoliating mask.

**Pro Tip(s):** "Earth Empress" Shakaya Leone, author of *Naked Beauty* (and all the ageless beauty inspiration you will ever need), suggests gently "pressing" rather than "scrubbing" your exfoliator into your skin. To do this, apply your exfoliator with a light palming motion. Ole Henriksen, founder of the eponymous skincare brand, suggests applying face oil prior to your scrub to act as an extra layer of protection for your skin. This is perfect if you love to scrub, but have sensitive skin or are prone to broken capillaries like I am.

## Step 4: Steam

Whether you are steaming using the old-fashioned towel-over-the-head method or you splurged on a fancy pro-style system, you will want a comfortable place to sit while you enjoy this pampering step. Adding flowers, herbs, and/or essential oil to your water will make it extra fancy, and I consider it an optional but awesome addition to the old-fashioned steam. Depending on your preference (I love rose, lavender, chamomile, and nettle), you can add a ½ cup of mixed dried flowers and/or several drops of essential oil to your steam.

**Old-fashioned Method:** Bring 3 cups of water to a boil and pour into a glass or ceramic bowl. Add your mixture of flowers, herbs, and essential oils, giving them a little stir. Drape a towel over your head to tent the steam in as you carefully lower your face directly over the steam (this should feel warm, not hot!).

**Fancy Facial Steam:** If you opt to use a home facial steam, you may have the option to add aromatherapy, as some models are designed with a separate container specifically for that purpose. To use your steamer, follow the manufacturer's directions.

Close your eyes, breathe deeply, and enjoy the steam for about 5 to 10 minutes depending on your sensitivity. Skin that flushes easily will want the least amount of time, while oily skin might want the most.

**Quick Tip:** While I love steam during my professional facials, sometimes I opt for a simpler steam during my home facials and fake it with a nice warm washcloth draped over my face until it cools.

**Pro Tip:** I love this tip from my friend Darcy Hunt, one of the "sages of beauty" at Sage Salon, my go-to spot for all things beauty in Napa, California. Your steam is the perfect time to gently massage exfoliating enzymes (or a product containing them) into your skin to boost their magical powers. To mix up enzymes, scoop them into a glass or ceramic bowl, then add a little water (or the activator it comes with) and stir with a spoon. Apply the enzymes to your face, neck, and décolleté and massage while you steam. Try this tip with a pro-style home facial steamer unless you're more coordinated than I am while draping a towel over your head.

**Step 4: Massage (my favorite part!)**

Not only is a facial massage wonderfully relaxing (even when you do it yourself), it also stimulates circulation and facial muscles while draining the lymph system of excess fluid. Different techniques have different effects on the skin: vigorous, upward movements are excellent for stimulating collagen and elastin production, while slow, gentle, upward strokes are good for lymphatic drainage. Both Beautycounter and Living Libations make exceptional face oils that are perfect for this step.

**Quick Tip:** If you don't have time to indulge in a longer face massage, a few passes with your gemstone roller will give you a nice circulation boost.

**Pro Tip:** This tip from Shelley is an absolute gem! Her unique "slap and tap" technique is designed to firm your skin through epidermal growth stimulation. It might look a little silly, but the result is healthy, energized skin (yes, please!). As she explains, "When we want to fluff a pillow we slap and tap it a bit and it plumps up. The same theory may be applied to your skin care routine. If you slap and tap your skin quickly and rhythmically you energize it, increasing the collagen and elastin production." Shelley does this during facials with her clients (it's my favorite part), then demonstrates how to do it at home as part of your daily routine. You can watch Shelley demonstrate the technique on her S4 Skincare YouTube channel ("How to firm your skin with the Slap + Tap technique").

**Step 5: Masks**

Now that you've cleansed, exfoliated, steamed, and massaged your face, it's perfectly primed to receive the nutrients in your facial mask. Wondering what mask to try? When deciding on a mask, take a good look at your skin and aim to choose a mask that addresses your main concern. Have more than one concern? Feel free to use different masks on different areas of your face. Whether it's deep cleansing, brightening, hydrating, or plumping you're after, there's a mask that addresses your specific needs. Just be sure to choose one from a company whose philosophy is in line with your intention to use the safest and most effective products you can get your hands on. Apply your mask according to the directions on the label and allow it to work its magic for the recommended time. Use a warm, wet washcloth to slowly massage the mask off your skin.

**Quick Tip:** If you're short on time, choose a mask with a shorter leave-on time. A lot can be done in just a minute or two!

**Pro Tip:** Sage Darcy suggests applying a hydrating serum under your mask to give your skin a pretty "plump" look for special occasions. I consider my weekly home facials just such an occasion, and this little tip works wonders! Look for a serum containing hyaluronic acid, which helps lock moisture into the skin.

### Step 6: Tone

Toners are beneficial for hydration, balancing the skin's pH and contracting pores. A good toner also helps other products to penetrate the skin. I love toners with botanicals, herbs, and essential oils and am currently pretty partial to rosewater. When purchasing a toner, keep in mind that despite marketing claims to tighten, soothe, and soften your skin, conventional toners are typically a chemical soup of alcohol, fragrance, parabens, and hydrogenated oils, so choose wisely.

**Quick Tip:** While toning is a pretty quick step in and of itself, you can be doing a lot more than refreshing your face when you choose a toner with active ingredients that target your particular skincare needs.

**Pro Tip:** My stint in Manhattan's (now trendy) Lower East Side coincided with the opening of the Christine Chin Spa. Dubbed "Mean Christine" for her thorough work and attention to detail (the extractions!), she set up shop a block from my apartment, so I was lucky enough to get personal attention from Christine herself before all the supermodels and fashion and beauty insiders made that nearly impossible. I wasn't a toner loyalist before getting schooled by Mean Christine, but she told me never to skip this simple step (she believes it gets rid of plaques on the skin). When you get beauty advice at this level, you just follow it.

**Step 7: Treat**

Treating your skin with a serum is such a great way to add concentrated, active ingredients to your skincare regime. Typically, a serum will be the thinnest product you apply, going on top of toned skin and penetrating quickly. Depending on your beauty wish list, you might try:

**Antioxidant:** neutralizes environmental free radicals that cause photo aging

**Hydrating:** delivers an extra layer of hydration and soothes irritated skin

**Exfoliating:** typically used at night, these work to dissolve dead skin cells

**Firming:** targets more advanced signs of living in your skin

**Brightening:** evens out skin tone and fades hyperpigmentation

Your serum likes to be sealed in with something that protects the skin barrier, so let it absorb and then move on to the following step.

**Quick Tip:** If your skin is sensitive, be sure you are applying your serum to thoroughly dry skin, as damp skin may absorb the active ingredients too quickly, causing irritation. If this isn't a concern for you, applying to damp skin is a nice way to boost the active ingredients.

**Pro Tip:** Sage Darcy gave me the brilliant tip of layering serums so that you get *all* the benefits you're after. Just be sure to use the most targeted one first so you don't dilute the actives and let the serums dry between layers. For evening, apply a rich moisturizer after your serum to lock in hydration. You'll wake up to super nourished, happy skin!

**Step 8: Moisturize**

This essential step seals the deal. I like to put a few drops of facial oil into the palm of my hand, lightly rub my hands together to distribute, and then gently press the oil into my skin before layering on a moisturizer. You might like that too.

**Quick Tip:** I can sometimes skip a daytime moisturizer after my facial oil and go straight to SPF. Since I favor a "no makeup" makeup look, my tinted SPF performs double duty.

**Pro Tip:** Shelley suggests applying moisturizer to your skin while it's still a bit damp from your serum to boost product penetration. Wait for everything to dry and apply your SPF for daytime.

### Bonus Step: Gemstone Facial Roller (Your New Best Friend)

An age-old tool used in Eastern beauty rituals, the gemstone facial roller is about to be your new best friend! While jade and rose quartz are arguably the most popular, there are a wide variety of gemstones being used for this purpose, so pick one that feels like an energetic match for you. Physically, these gemstones increase blood circulation, aid lymphatic drainage (bye-bye puffy eyes), promote cell turnover, and improve elasticity. Regular use of a gemstone roller gives you an immediate beauty boost and bonus beauty benefits as you slow the progression of wrinkles. It's super easy to use—start at the center of your neck and move the gemstone roller across your skin in upward and outward motions. Aim to roll for about two minutes. If you notice a little flush, that's circulation increasing to help you get your glow on!

**Cool Tip:** Your gemstone roller is a master multitasker that you can use throughout each step of your facial to help your product absorb better (even your mask). It's perfect to de-puff sleepy eyes in the morning, and storing it in your refrigerator is a cool tip. I love to spritz a bit of rosewater or other hydrosol over my face and give my skin a few passes with my gemstone roller for a quick pick-me-up any time of day—so refreshing!

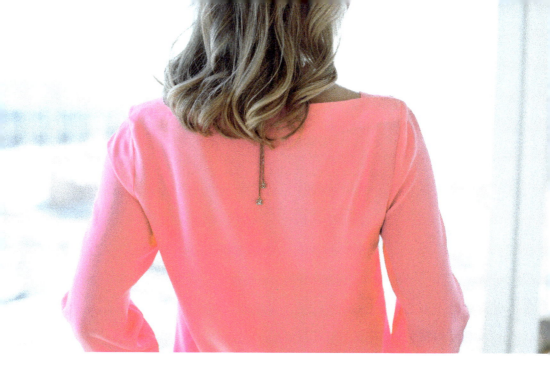

*"The loose strands of a beautiful woman don't have to be combed."*
— Rumi

## Beauty Secrets from Head to Toe: That Pretty Head of Yours

Everybody loves a good hair day, but often the products we use are loaded with toxic chemicals that have the potential to affect our cells, tissues, and organs; and the water we wash our hair with can be an issue too. Our hair follicles are rich in blood vessels close to the scalp. When we wash our hair, the warm water opens up these follicles, making it easy for the ingredients in our hair-care products and water to be absorbed by our system. Ideally, consider investing in a home water filtration system. If that isn't possible, installing a water filter for your showerhead is an excellent choice to minimize your exposure to chemicals and chlorine found in tap water. To make a safer choice, be on the lookout for:

**Sulfates:** Sulfates like sodium lauryl sulfate (SLS) and sodium laureth sulfate (SLES) are chemicals commonly used in shampoo, oven cleaners, and other products to create a foaming action. Known endocrine disrupters and suspected carcinogens, both SLS and SLES are classified as toxic and harmful on the EWG's Skin Deep Database.

**Formaldehyde:** Used as a preservative, formaldehyde irritates the skin and can cause allergies, joint pain, inflammation, dizziness, and chronic fatigue. It is also a known carcinogen.

**Fragrance:** Though companies are required by law to list the ingredients that make up their products, the word "Fragrance" is considered a trade secret, so companies aren't legally bound to disclose what chemicals they use to create a scent. Dozens or even hundreds of chemicals can be involved in a fragrance formulation, so this is an ingredient we need to be super mindful about.

**DEA, MEA & TEA:** Commonly found in shampoos, soaps, bubble bath, and facial wash, the chemicals Diethanolamine (DEA), Monoethanolamine (MEA), and Triethanolamine (TEA) are known hormone disrupters and irritants.

**Ethyl & Isopropyl Alcohols:** These petroleum-based alcohols are found in many products as a solvent or surfactant (antifreeze, paints, and varnishes to name a few). Used in hair products, these toxins are drying to the hair shaft and can lead to scalp irritation and hair breakage.

**PEG:** Commonly used as an emulsifier, Polyethylene Glycol (PEG) contains high amounts of heavy metals known to cause neurological, autoimmune, and kidney issues.

Speaking of good hair days, it can be simpler than you think. Your happy, healthy hair loves:

**Drying Naturally:** Let your hair dry naturally whenever possible, and limit hairdryers and styling tools to special occasions.

**Being Dirty:** Over-washing can strip your hair of its natural oils, so try to let your hair get a little dirty between shampoos.

**Circulation:** Scalp massage helps boost blood flow in the head and neck area, improving hair growth and relaxing the nervous system (bonus points for using essential oil).

## Stimulating Scalp Massage = Bliss Inducing + Circulation Boosting + Unique to You

Your happy, healthy hair loves circulation, and you will love the bliss-inducing side effects!

## You Will Need:

- 3 drops essential oil of your choosing
- 1 teaspoon carrier oil of your choosing

## Make It Your Own: Essential Oil

**Chamomile:** A calming little flower from the daisy family, chamomile soothes a dry or sensitive scalp while boosting softness and sheen.

**Clary Sage:** Known to be particularly helpful for female pattern baldness, it is said to provide a balancing effect on hormones.

**Lavender:** This well-established folk remedy moisturizes the scalp, balances sebum production, and soothes your nerves, making it pretty much perfect.

**Rosemary:** The revitalizing properties of rosemary give you the perfect combination of shiny, bouncy hair *and* a mood boost.

**Ylang Ylang:** Native to tropical Asia, this fragrant oil is traditionally used to stimulate and encourage hair growth. A massage with ylang ylang oil can ease tension headaches, ease anxiety, and encourage restful sleep.

**Make It Your Own: Carrier Oil**

**You Have Fine, Thin Hair:** Sunflower, coconut, grapeseed, olive, almond, or jojoba will give you bounce and volume.

**You Have Thick, Coarse Hair:** Avocado, olive, hemp, rosehip, sesame, or almond will add happy hydration.

**How-to:**

Once you've picked your essential and carrier oils, the measurements above can be used as a general guideline (you may need more or less). Starting at the front of the scalp and working towards the back, you can begin to massage your head freestyle, or using an "effleurage" (circular, stroking movements) or "petrissage" (gentle kneading). Massage gently but firmly and with a consistent pressure. For the most bliss-inducing experience, remain mindful of your breath and do some long deep breathing to increase the oxygen flow throughout your body. For an extra lovely treat, leave the oils to sit for a bit (even overnight) after you have completed your massage. At your leisure, wash and enjoy the benefits of your happy, healthy hair!

# Beauty Secrets from Head to Toe: Your Pearly Whites

*"Our gums and teeth are living tissue, and we should approach them a little differently than we would scrub a countertop ... most toothpastes and rinses, including many of the brands sold in health food stores, use chemical and synthetic ingredients that are more appropriate for industrial purposes than for cleaning*

*the delicate tissue of the body or cultivating oral health. Brushing with these chemicals may be harmful to our health."*

— Nadine Artemis, author of *Successful Self-Dentistry*

If what you've been brushing your pearly whites with has a big fat warning label that reads "May Be Harmful If Swallowed," believe it. The foamy experience you get with commercial toothpaste is thanks to detergents and surfactants like sodium laureth sulfate and sodium lauryl sulfate; known skin irritants, hormone and endocrine disruptors, and suspected carcinogens. While you likely aren't purposefully eating gobs of toothpaste, the rate of absorption in the mouth is very high. As Timothy A. Kersten, DDS, puts it, "The blood that runs through your tooth will run through your toe in one minute." Luckily, a dry toothbrush with a dab of salt, baking soda, or a pure botanical serum like neem or peppermint does everything you want your toothpaste to do, but without the potential to harm you in the process. As more and more studies highlight the relationship between poor oral health and conditions like inflammation, diabetes, and even heart disease, now is the perfect time to consider upgrading the way you care for your pearly whites (your whole body thanks you!).

## Open Wide—What Do You See?

If you have a mouth full of silver amalgam fillings, consider having them removed by a biologically trained dentist. Silver-mercury amalgam has been used as a filling material for well over a century, and while it has enjoyed the reputation of being an inexpensive, long-lasting tooth filling, mercury vapor is a huge source of toxicity. Mercury vaporizes off the amalgam fillings 24/7. Mercury also infuses into the pulp chamber of the tooth and enters the bloodstream. Based on a number of studies in Sweden, the World Health Organization review of inorganic mercury in 1991 determined that mercury absorption is estimated to be approximately four times higher from amalgam fillings than from fish consumption. If that's something that concerns you, be sure to check out my resources for finding a biologically trained dentist in your area in chapter seven.

## Tongue Scraping = Bacteria Busting + Breath Freshening + Taste Bud Enhancing

I was fascinated when I learned that a tool for reducing food cravings was the Ayurvedic tradition of tongue scraping. When the mouth can still taste the food, you may end up experiencing cravings for foods previously eaten. It also reverses the process of desensitizing your taste buds, which happens to most people to a greater or lesser extent as we age. When old residue is removed from the tongue, it allows you to taste more subtle flavors in food. Scraping your tongue also prevents bad breath, especially for people who eat a lot of dairy and build up mucus in the mouth, nose, and throat.

**You Will Need:**

- tongue scraper (the back of a spoon works in a pinch)

**How-to:**

After brushing and flossing your teeth, gently place the tongue scraper as far back on your tongue as you comfortably can and scrape forward several times, making sure you've covered all the surface area and sides of your tongue. Don't worry if this makes you gag a little bit—that reflex actually helps strengthen the connection between your brain and your gut (good to know, right?). Continue scraping until there is no white residue left on the scraper, and remember to rinse it thoroughly under hot water. Tongue scrapers are readily available at the pharmacy, your local health food store, or online.

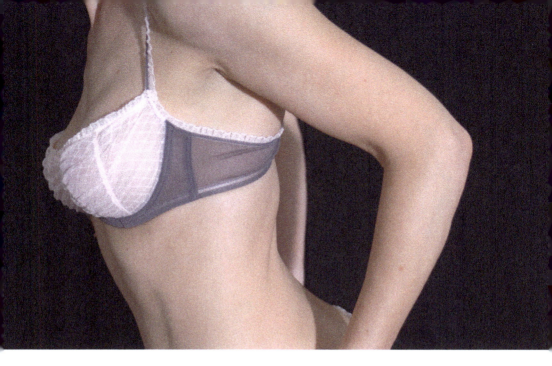

> "These cherished, tender tissues that embody both sensuality and sustenance have, for many, become a burden ... There is an estrogenic-epidemic in our erogenous zone, and our breasts are reacting; worldwide, every 23 seconds a woman is diagnosed with breast cancer."
>
> — Nadine Artemis, *Renegade Beauty*

## Beauty Secrets from Head to Toe: Your Perfectly Imperfect Breasts

Every 23 seconds a woman is diagnosed with breast cancer, and like many of you, breast health is a deeply personal issue for me. Mama Ruth's sisters have both struggled with a breast cancer diagnosis, and while my Aunt Pat has experienced a full recovery since her diagnosis more than a decade ago, my Aunt Linda's breast cancer metastasized and she is now living with stage-4 bone cancer. My initial response to the breast cancer in my family was fear. Fear for both of my aunts, fear of Mama Ruth being diagnosed, and fear of my own dense and fibrocystic breasts. I fed that fear by having every lump and bump examined (sometimes biopsied) and anxiously awaiting my own cancer diagnosis.

The energy of fear did little to support my intention of living in vibrant health, but stumbling upon David Wolfe's interview "What Every Woman Needs to Know" with Nadine Artemis did. Losing her own mother to breast cancer in 2014, Nadine spoke about the importance of avoiding "bad estrogen" dominance, the hidden dangers of mammograms, and why underwire bras contribute to breast health issues by restricting the lymphatic system. Empowered with new information, I worked with my functional medicine doctor to check my hormone levels and traded in my mammograms for breast thermography. I also committed to taking the following daily steps to support my breast health:

**I Ditched My Bra:** These days I consider wearing a bra more of a special occasion thing than a daily ritual. The health of our lymphatic system is intimately connected to our breasts, and when they are trapped inside an underwire bra all day, it can impede our body's natural removal of fluids. Look for red marks on your skin after removing your bra, and if you find them, know that it's time to consider wearing no bra, a softer bra, or a yoga top. If that's too much to consider, you can start by going bra-free at home. Also, if you're reluctant to give up your bra because you fear it will lead to sagging, you'll be happy to know that's a myth. A 15-year French study found that women who went braless for a year actually received a welcome lift, as well as fading of stretch marks and overall firmer breasts.

**I Ditched My Deodorant:** Instead of applying aluminum and parabens to my armpits, I generally opt to go without, and when that's not a good option, I use a nontoxic deodorant. Sealing off one of the body's primary toxin-releasing areas with chemicals is just a bad idea, and while studies connecting antiperspirants and deodorants to cancer are inconclusive, a lot of breast cancer is found in the armpit. It's also been discovered that 99% of breast cancer tissue has parabens in it. I won't lie, some nontoxic deodorants don't *actually* work, but these ones do: the Poetic Pits line from Nadine Artemis (livinglibations.

com) and the wide variety of products available from Primal Pit Paste (primalpitpaste.com).

**I Jump Bra-Free:** You already know I'm a huge fan of rebounding on a mini trampoline, and for breast health, I do this without any additional support. I admit I had to be talked into this one because the idea of bouncing up and down without a bra wasn't super appealing to me *or* my size-32D breasts! I eased my way into the practice by doing the Health Bounce while intermittently supporting my breasts with my hands and then bouncing freely. As I got used to it, I spent way less time holding my breasts, and by the time I started jumping without any support, I was delighted to find that my once often-tender breasts were noticeably less so after incorporating this into my routine.

**I Massage My Breasts:** Breast massage is a hugely regenerative practice that stimulates both the lymphatic and circulatory system, allowing fresh blood and fluids to flow in, and toxins to flow out. It loosens up tight breast muscles and stimulates the endocrine system to secrete a powerful cocktail of youthful hormones (yes, please!). Over time, massaging the breasts may also support the elasticity of the ligaments in the chest, providing improved breast support.

The best tool you have for breast health is your own awareness of your body. Whether large, small, round, tubular, proportionate, asymmetrical, with big or small areolas, or flat or protruding nipples, our breasts are as beautiful and individual as each of us. The best way to honor your own perfectly imperfect breasts is to become intimately familiar with them, and having a regular breast massage practice is the perfect way to do this. Performing breast massage with essential oil is a really lovely practice that can be performed at any point during the menstrual cycle (depending on your comfort). Our breasts are considered our love center because they sit on either side of our heart and represent the external expression of our heart chi.

**You Will Need:**

- your bare breasts
- essential oil (I love Living Libations' breast massage oil or rose otto)
- carrier oil of your choice (coconut oil is particularly nice)
- a soft inner smile

**How-to:**

This practice begins with a smile, which I think is sweet. First, warm your hands by rubbing them together vigorously, and as you do this, set the intention that your practice will bring love and health to your breasts. Next, combine your carrier and essential oils in the palm of your hand, and then place your hands on the center of your chest. Cultivate a soft inner smile to your breasts as you take several long deep breaths. Begin massaging inward and upward in a circular motion, slowly covering the entire chest. Continue to massage slowly and gently for about 2 to 5 minutes. As you massage, keep in mind that your breast tissue extends from the breastbone in the center of the chest to the underarms and from below the collarbone down to the sixth or seventh rib. Use the time spent performing your breast massage to become familiar with how your breasts feel, and if you notice changes that concern you, be sure to reach out to a health-care professional.

# Beauty Rituals from Head to Toe: Your Lovely Lady Bits

> *"The vagina, the savory peach, the fertile crescent of our femininity, is not merely the reproductive plumbing that reductionist science would have us believe. Neither are the jewels of the nether region a receptacle. The vagina is, in fact, a gateway and passage to the brain, the body, and the spirit. It is also a sublime portal where the form and formlessness of a soul can coalesce."*
>
> — Nadine Artemis, *Renegade Beauty*

In *Renegade Beauty*, Nadine Artemis writes that the American Congress of Obstetricians and Gynecologists cautions that women seeking "designer vaginas" should be informed about the lack of data supporting the efficacy of these procedures and their potential complications, including infection, altered sensation, adhesions, and scarring. This warning coincides with an increase in the plastic surgeries of labiaplasty, vaginoplasty and revirgination. Ancient Taoist and Tantric texts revered the vagina as a source of wisdom connected to the True Self, and as such, it must be treated with care and respect. With this in mind, I invite you to care for your own lovely lady bits in a way that honors, rather than shames, your True Self.

## Upgrade Your Feminine Hygiene

Commercial feminine hygiene products contain various substances, including rayon, which is derived from wood treated with chlorine. Chlorine bleaching produces the chemical commonly known as dioxin, which is classified as a "known human carcinogen" by the World Health Organization. Monthly use of these products amounts to significant repeated exposure. To be on the safe side, ditch your potentially harmful feminine hygiene products in favor of these:

- Organic tampons & pads
- Cotton (reusable) pads
- The Keeper (reusable, natural rubber)

## Your Feminine Essence: Clues to Health

Diet, digestion, and hydration all play a role in the scent (and flavor) of our vaginal secretions. The natural scent of your vagina can tell you a lot about the health of your body. When your inner ecology is out of balance, this is communicated to you through changing (and often stronger or foul-smelling) odor. Disguising these clues to health through the use of fragrant sprays or douches is just a bad idea. Not only does it prevent us from healing, these products contain ingredients that can potentially make matters worse. Rather than relying on questionable and potentially toxic products, consider becoming curious about your not-so-fresh feeling. Here's a start:

**Your Diet:** Like the rest of your body, your vagina benefits from your choice of eating an organic whole foods diet with plenty of greens and limited sugar (candida loves sugar). Already doing this? Try adding more fermented foods, oral doses of lactobacillus bifidus, and a probiotic to increase your friendly flora.

**Read Labels:** The ingredients you avoid in your skincare are the same ingredients you want to avoid when caring for your lady bits. More permeable than our skin, the mucous membranes in the vagina absorb what you put on and in it quickly. Your vagina is a self-cleaning organism, so a nice rinse with warm water is all the extra help she really needs.

**Rethink Your Contraceptive:** Similar to antibiotics, birth control pills reduce colonies of good microflora, contributing to imbalance (think yeast infections and bacterial vaginosis).

**Personal Grooming:** Grooming is a personal preference, but keep in mind that waxing and shaving can inflame hair follicles and leave microscopic open wounds. Combined with a naturally moist environment, this can create the perfect breeding ground for bacteria to grow. If you go this route, a bit of soothing, antibacterial coconut oil is perfect for your aftercare.

**Go Commando:** Like you, your vagina likes to breathe and she hates polyester. If she's constantly covered in panties, her natural moistness can lead to itching, irritation, and yeast overgrowth. If going commando isn't your daily preference, try sleeping sans panties and opt for cotton undergarments most of the time.

**Send Love:** Our emotional well-being is a key factor in the health of our vaginas. In her book *Emergence of the Sensual Woman: Awakening Our Erotic Innocence*, Dr. Saida Desilets writes that "if we experience cramps or other physical pain in our genitals we can take a moment to stop everything we are doing and just rest. Placing our hands on our heart we begin to feel love grow there. Smiling to our heart until it is warm and soft, we can then bring this warm, loving energy down to our genitals by smiling down at them." I think this is such a beautiful practice (you will too).

While many imbalances can be corrected in the early stages, it's always wise to consult a health-care professional if you are experiencing an unpleasant odor, pain, or discomfort.

## Little Miss Sunshine = Balancing + Healing + Slightly Scandalous

The ancient Taoist practice of yoni "sunning" is about shining light on dark spaces. It is believed that by exposing the darkest or most yin part of our bodies to yang sunlight, we bring harmony and balance to our energy system. We do this by allowing our yonis to drink in the sunshine (yes, really).

**You Will Need:**

- a sunny day
- a bit of privacy (a backyard is perfect, but a sunny window will do)
- a towel, blanket, or cushion to lie on

**How-to:**

Lie on your back with your feet together, knees falling to opposite sides like a butterfly. Position yourself so that you can feel the warmth of the sun enter your yoni. Bring your hands to an inverted "V" on your womb, outlining your pubic triangle. Take a few long deep breaths into your yoni. With every inhale, invite love and gratitude, and with your exhale, allow any tightness or tension to melt into the earth beneath you. On your next inhale imagine sipping in the life-force energy of the sun into your yoni. At the top of the inhale, hold your breath and contract your PC muscle (as if you are trying not to pee) and begin massaging the womb area in a slow circular motion. As you massage, imagine spreading the healing light of the sun's energy throughout your yoni. On your exhale, allow old energies to be released back into the earth. Continue this practice, inhaling light and exhaling dark, for five minutes. When finished, allow your breath to return to its normal pattern and rest for a time.

## Beauty Rituals from Head to Toe: Heavenly Hands + Fabulous Feet

> *"Forget not that the earth delights to feel your bare feet and the winds long to play with your hair."*
> — Kahlil Gibran

I've always loved a mani pedi (especially with Mama Ruth by my side), but conventional nail polish and the chemicals we use to remove them are a toxic shitstorm. Nail polishes often include:

**Toluene:** A chemical known to cause reproductive harm, it is also found in gasoline and the CDC warns that it can cause central nervous system problems.

**Formaldehyde:** For starters, it preserves dead things, and you, my dear, are a living breathing human. Formaldehyde is a known carcinogen, and when used in lab preparations, it comes with strict warnings to avoid inhalation or skin contact.

**Dibutyl phthalate (DBP):** Banned in Europe because it is known to cause reproductive problems, the Environmental

Working Group classifies DBP at the highest danger level and warns that it can cause organ problems and endocrine disruption.

I consider polish a special occasion kind of thing and like that we have a lot more options for better beauty these days. If you've been using conventional polish and would like to make a switch, there are options with safer ratings on the Environment Working Group database (ewg.org).

**Fresh Start Soak = Cuticle Softening + Nail Strengthening + Stain Busting**

This is the perfect fresh start if you are weaning off polish and notice your natural nails aren't ready for prime time. The lemon and baking soda will go to work on any yellowing (it happens), while sea salt softens cuticles and strengthens your nails. Use the recipe below for soaking hands and double it for soaking your toes.

**You Will Need:**

- a soaking bowl
- a nailbrush
- ¼ cup warm water
- ¼ cup lemon juice
- 1 teaspoon baking soda
- 1 teaspoon sea salt
- a bit of coconut oil for after your soak

**How-to:**

Mix ingredients in a small or large bowl, then soak nails for about 10 minutes. After soaking, use your nailbrush to scrub away any tougher stains. Dry your hands and then rub a bit of coconut oil into your nail beds. This simple cuticle cream strengthens your nails and smells delicious!

## Barefoot Beauty = Energizing + Health Promoting + Mood Boosting + Pain Reducing

While Clinton Ober, a cable systems engineering entrepreneur turned biohacker, was the first to uncover the health benefits of a simple practice called "Earthing," your body always knew. There are in fact so many benefits to being a barefoot beauty that Mr. Ober and his colleagues, Dr. Steve Sinatra and Martin Zucker, wrote a fascinating book called *Earthing: The Most Important Health Discovery Ever!* (give it a read). The book reveals the background to what is considered by many to be a new healing paradigm. The basic theory is that our bodies develop a positive charge that is slowly dispelled when we touch the Earth, whose negatively charged electrons balance this accumulation. The result is that you not only *feel* grounded (because you are), but your body is in the ideal state to create optimal health.

**You Will Need:**

- your bare feet
- access to the Earth (grass, gravel, dirt, sand, or concrete)

**How-to:**

Walk, stand, or sit barefoot on the ground for a half hour or so as often as possible, daily being ideal. If the ideal isn't doable, Earthing has taken a decidedly high-tech turn and you can now get yourself all manner of Earthing gear from earthing.com (Mama Ruth swears by the fitted sheets).

# Beauty Secrets from Head to Toe: The Naked Truth

*"Love your body. Be kind to it, nourish it, tender it. It is the pure instrument of expression that allows you to experience life on this plane."*
— Ramtha

Every inch of the one and only you is covered in skin, so feeling comfortable in it matters (a lot). If you've been nourishing your body with foods it loves and enjoying any of the self-care practices I shared in previous chapters, you're likely already noticing a healthy glow to your skin. If you haven't given yourself that opportunity yet and loving the skin you're in is one of your intentions, feel free to start right here, right now. Since health and beauty are besties, every step you take toward creating a more vibrant, healthy you will be rewarded with improved skin from head to toe.

## Cellulite, Stretch Marks & Jiggly Bits

If the beauty industry has convinced you that your cellulite is a problem, then they've done their job, which is to sell expensive cellulite-banishing lotions and potions to the 80% of women who have this "problem" (same goes for your stretch marks and jiggly bits). Nadine Artemis reminds us that women are energy-storage experts and that cellulite is part of our expert fat-storage capacity (it's handy for birthing babes). While cellulite is a normal condition of being a woman, when our systems are out of balance, it tends to show up on our skin. The naked truth is that there are no quick fixes, but there *are* steps you can take to start feeling more comfortable in your skin. Here are some of my favorites:

> **Clean Up Your Body Care:** If you've cleaned up your beauty act by switching to clean cosmetics (yay, you!) but are still using conventional products in and out of your shower, now's the perfect time to make a healthier choice. Make the

commitment to using safer products from head to toe and your whole body will thank you.

**Filter Your Water:** The Environmental Working Group spent three years investigating the country's drinking water. What they found was that roughly 85% of the population was using water that contained over 300 contaminants, more than half of which aren't regulated by the EPA. Among the cocktail of contaminants coming from municipal tap water is fluoride, which has been shown to disrupt collagen (not good news for the skin you're in). If your budget allows, installing a whole-house water filtration system is ideal. If that isn't feasible, individual drinking water and shower filter units are a worthwhile health and beauty investment.

**Boost Your Collagen:** When our youthful collagen levels are at their peak, skin is smooth, firm, and vibrant. As collagen production slows around age 30, this natural aging process gives skin its more lived-in look (think sagging and wrinkles). It also allows fat cells the room to poke through the connective tissue, accentuating the appearance of cellulite. Boosting collagen production and reducing the collagen degradation that occurs from chronic stress, hormone imbalance, or poor lifestyle choices may be helpful in the reduction of cellulite. Increasing your consumption of foods high in vitamin C will help the amino acids lysine and proline convert to collagen, while healing bone broth helps build connective tissue, making skin smoother (less cellulite, fewer wrinkles) and healthier.

**Move Your Lymph:** Excess fluid in connective tissue can cause visible swelling of thighs, hips, and abdomen, accentuating the appearance of cellulite. Improved circulation from daily movement will keep the skin and connective tissue healthy by speeding up the elimination of waste and excess fluid. Finding ways to get moving in your daily life is key. Bonus points for adding dry brushing to your skin-loving routine (I show you how below).

**Take a Bath:** A recent study published in the journal of *Temperature* found that an hour-long soak in hot water produced similar anti-inflammatory and blood sugar responses as 60 minutes of moderate activity and burns as many calories as a half-hour walk. Consider this self-care staple your new workout. The "Bathe in Love" ritual at the end of this chapter is the perfect start.

**Get Naked:** If you spend most of your time avoiding your naked reflection in the mirror, you may need to ease into this one (I promise, it's worth it). Being naked not only gives skin a chance to fully breathe (which it loves), but it can actually help you learn to love the skin you're in. One study by *A Journal of Happiness Studies* found that by simply spending more time naked, an individual can increase their body image, self-esteem, and life satisfaction. Try sleeping naked to ease into the nudnik thing and work your way up to solo naked dance parties. While you're at it, see other people naked too (airbrushed media images don't count). It will help you let go of any preconceived ideas of what naked bodies "should". look like and appreciate the unique beauty of the human body.

**Love Yourself Anyway:** The best treatment for stretch marks, cellulite, and jiggly bits is to learn to love your body just as it is. Next time you find yourself thinking critical thoughts about your body, take a long deep breath and on the exhale whisper "I love you right there" to whatever body part needs it the most.

## Dry Skin Brushing = Circulation Boosting + Exfoliating + Lymph Moving

While learning to love the one and only you is the best treatment for cellulite, stretch marks, and jiggly bits, having a solid self-care routine is *also* a good plan. Dry brushing is an excellent place to start!

Truly the best part of my morning routine, I use my time spent dry brushing as an opportunity to check in with my naked self, then tailor my routine and products to best support my ever-changing needs. There are several brushes on the market intended for this purpose, and while a lot of it comes down to personal preference, look for a brush made from natural fibers and start with a not-too-stiff brush.

**You Will Need:**

- a dry skin brush
- essential oil (optional, but awesome)

**How-to:** If you want to incorporate essential oil, put a few drops in the palm of your hand and run the dry brush over it a couple of times. This is my favorite time to use the Living Libations "CelluLight" oil on the spots that want more circulation. Beginning with the soles of your feet, work the brush in upward circular movements, always in the direction of your heart. Continue brushing, moving to the tops of the feet, the calves, and the thighs. Move to the back and remember to brush in the direction of the heart, alternating sides, as you brush your booty, lower back, and sides. Moving back to the front, use circular counterclockwise strokes on the abdomen to encourage healthy digestion. Lightly brush your breasts in a figure-8 motion. Reach around and brush your upper back. Proceed to your hands and arms. Once you've finished brushing, take a moment to admire your rosy glow and feel the increased energy circulating in your body!

**Beauty Note:** If you decide to use an essential oil with your dry brush, it's often recommended to shower first so that you don't waste those precious (sometimes pricey) oils. That said, I like to make my own rules, so I use a bit of circulation-boosting essential oil on areas I think might like that both before *and* after my shower or bath. You can make your own rules too.

# Sing Your Soul Song

The summer I turned 11 Mama Ruth and I moved into a converted loft in an old creamery in Bodega, California. Rustic and hip before its time, the creamery was the kind of space my adult self would consider charming and a lucky find. My 11-year-old self found it more weird than charming, but the claw-foot bathtub made up for it, and that was *before* I met my frog friend. It is believed that when a frog appears it's time to sing your soul song, and while that may or may not be true, when a tiny frog travels through the pipes and perches himself on the ledge of your bathtub, it does make your soul sing (he did this for years). Frog became my daily companion, keeper of my secrets, witness to my soul song.

When Mama Ruth and I moved from the creamery to a converted barn in the Bodega town center, our (somewhat) fancier digs offered a more modern vibe with a standard issue shower-over-tub. I tried the new tub, but it wasn't the same. I missed my beloved claw-foot, the warm embrace of its smooth porcelain, the sturdy feel of its feet on the ground, and the way it kept my water hot for as long as I needed. Mostly, I missed my frog. Most often I'd opt for a quick shower, and as time went by I let the memory of Frog fade. It would be decades later that I would meet Mud Pie and come to understand that your soul song never truly leaves you; she patiently waits for you to be ready to remember her words.

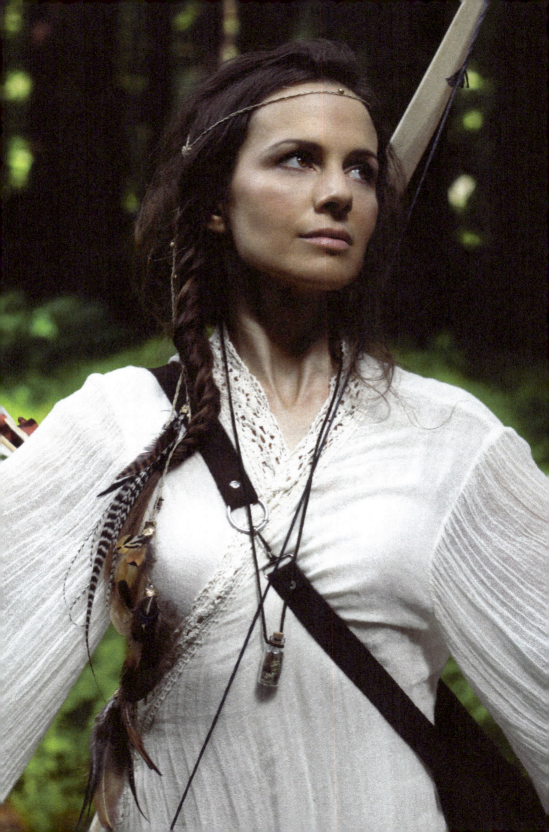

> *"It is my belief that the energy we put into something can be felt, and I'm passionate about putting more love out into the world. So, my making process always involves rituals that get me into a feeling space of joy, pleasure, gratitude and love before I begin and while I am creating. It keeps the process highly enjoyable and I think it is tasted and felt in the products I make. I hope you agree!"*
>
> — Rosalyn (Mud Pie) Fay, creator of the "Redwood Rose" line of rose-based handcrafted goods (rosalynfay.com)

## Mud Pie Magic

Before Rosalyn Fay (aka Mud Pie) ditched her city life like her *actual* life depended on it (it did), before she embarked on an epic healing journey that brought her back to her roots (and the dirt), and before she began crafting her rose-based magical goods in her Redwood Rose tiny house especially for *you*, she was the founder of True Colors TV—an inspirational video network created by women for women. In 2011 the Universe conspired to put Mud Pie on my (naked) path. We met on the set of the Women Enough BARE Campaign—a global event focused on promoting diversity in advertising, inspiring body confidence, and using the transformative power of storytelling to impact change. Unexpectedly, that day marked a shift in the focus of my own healing journey as I witnessed the wounds of my past showing up in my present self. Rosalyn had captured the part of me still silenced by shame, afraid to share the full truth of her story. More importantly, she captured the glimmer of hope that I would one day reclaim my voice and that my healing would allow me to step more powerfully into my work of supporting other women on their journey. That Mud Pie would someday homestead her little gypsy cabin-on-wheels just a frog's hop away from the very town I grew up in is all I need to believe in magic.

**Beauty Bonus: Mud Pie's Bathe in Love Ritual**

I was delighted when Mud Pie agreed to share her Bathe in Love Ritual with me (you will be too). This ritual is perfect for cultivating self-love and may even help you remember your own soul song.

**You Will Need:**

- a mixing bowl
- 4 cups Epsom salt
- rose absolute essential oil
- dried or fresh rose petals
- your heartfelt intention to love the one and only *you*

**How-to:** Set all ingredients out on a table and pour your salt into a mixing bowl. Take several long deep breaths as you consider what energy would best support your intention to cultivate self-love. Heart opening, forgiveness, pleasure or release are just some of possibilities, the key being to align yourself with an energy that most resonates for you. Feel into the qualities you desire, and as you are in the feeling state, add a couple drops of essential oil. With your hands, slowly mix it in with the salts, infusing the mixture with your feeling energy and ensuring the oils get evenly distributed. Imagine the energy of your intention coming from your heart out your hands and into the salts. If you like more scent, add a few more drops until it has the desired amount of fragrance, keeping in mind that Rose Absolute is concentrated so a little goes a long way. Next, add in the rose petals. Again feel your intention and infuse the mixture with it. As your bathwater is filling up, scoop out two cups of the salts and sprinkle it throughout the water, imagining all that good energy going into your bath. The final step is to get in and simply open to the experience. Feel your skin absorbing the loving energy of the rose surrounding you. I like to imagine I'm being cradled in the center of a rose in full bloom (you might like that too).

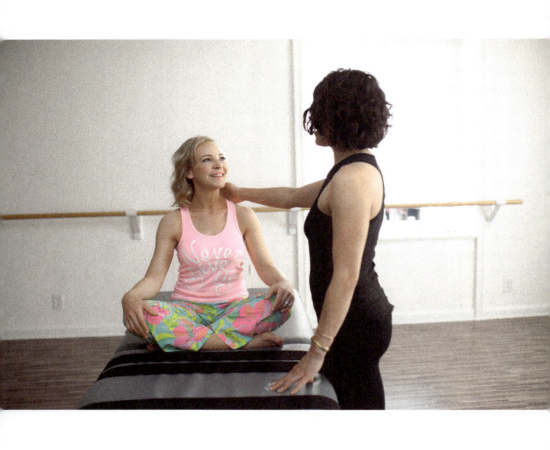

# CHAPTER SEVEN
# *Your* Path to Vibrant Health & Radiant Beauty

*"I have a vision for the kind of person I want to be, and I strive to live from and into that place. Sometimes, I transcend my impulses and become that. Other times, I suck. But I always try."*
— Brendon Burchard

**Each chapter of** this book has been an opportunity to share my healing journey with you, my personal path to vibrant health and radiant beauty. The first step on that path was my clear intention to honor my human body, and every step from there has been an attempt to live into that intention. This means that I greet each day with the conscious choice to meet myself exactly where I am with all the compassion and grace I can muster. Healing can be found in the smallest daily steps toward caring for the one and only you. The details of those steps are entirely up to you!

## Creating Your Intention

While I was attending the Institute for Integrative Nutrition, I had the great fortune of having Debbie Ford, the late bestselling author of *The Dark Side of the Light Chasers* and founder of the Institute for Integrative Coaching, as a guest teacher. Her message about embracing a vision of yourself at your best and then developing the qualities that will take you there, was so timely for me that I went on to read every single book she authored and continue to gift *The Best Year of Your Life: Dream It, Plan It, Live It* to my coaching clients. It was through Debbie's teachings that I came to understand the true magic of intention setting, which lies in its ability to support you in taking daily actions that are consistent with your vision for change.

A simple but powerful tool that we learned in nutrition school is called the "Circle of Life," and it's a wonderful starting point for getting clear on what areas in your life need the most attention (clarity and intentions go hand in hand). You'll need your journal, a writing instrument, and your dear brave heart.

The Circle of Life has 12 sections. Begin by drawing a large circle and place a small dot in the center of your circle. Next, divide your circle into twelve sections (like a pie), each representing the following areas of your well-being: spirituality, creativity, finances, career, education, health, physical activity, home cooking, home environment, relationships, social life, and joy. Look at each section of the Circle of Life and place a dot on the line marking how satisfied you are with each area of your life. A dot placed at the center of the circle or close to the middle indicates dissatisfaction, while a dot placed on the periphery indicates ultimate happiness. When you have placed a dot on each of the lines, connect the dots to see your Circle of Life. This will give you a clear visual of any imbalances and a starting point for creating your intention.

Now that you've focused in on the areas of your life that feel out of balance, it's time to turn inward and listen to what your own wise body has to tell you. Keep your journal handy and begin by closing your eyes, placing both hands over your heart, and taking several long deep breaths. As you tune in to your own heartbeat, feel as if you are breathing into the area surrounding your heart. As you continue to do this, bring to mind the areas of your life that are out of balance. If you begin to feel any fear or anxiety coming up for you, identify where in your body these feelings originate and simply whisper "I love you right there" as you imagine a golden light softening those emotions.

Continue long deep breathing and ask your heart which area is most important for you to focus on right now. Wait for your heart's answer, and when your starting point is clear, ask your heart what would need to be true for you to find balance in this area. Maybe your area of focus is physical activity, and moving your body more would allow you to find more balance; what would need to be true for you to move your body more? Could it be scheduling workouts on your calendar or asking a friend to join you at a yoga class? Or, maybe your focus is joy. What would need to be true for you to create more joy in your life? Trust your inner knowing to guide you to the answer.

Now, grab your journal and write your little heart out! There is no right or wrong way to do this. Writing helps connect you to your intuition, allowing you to listen to what your body, mind and spirit need to thrive. Listen and write it down. Write for at least 15 minutes to give yourself time to get going, and afterward, sit and see how you feel. When you're ready, begin reading the message. This love letter from your own wise and wonderful heart will lead you to your intention (I promise). When we tune in to the wisdom of our own hearts, magic happens!

## It Starts With You, but You Don't Have to Go It Alone

I feel honored to have worked with some amazing wellness practitioners over the years. While each has their own unique perspective and approach to healing, the common thread amongst them is their dedication to teaching me to listen to my body and intuition to understand what I need to heal. When seeking out the support of a qualified wellness practitioner, it's helpful to be both open to new ways of approaching your health, and to find a practitioner whose philosophy is in line with your own beliefs about healing.

While there are a variety of websites that offer listings of trained practitioners in your area, many qualified practitioners are not on any professional websites or lists. Connecting with others in your community and getting word-of-mouth recommendations is a great way to find practitioners aligned with your personal definition of optimum health. We are bio-individuals with unique needs, and the support we seek on this path should be unique as well. If you feel inspired to be supported on your path to vibrant health and radiant beauty, but don't know where to start, consider this your quick-start guide.

## Health Coaching: What It Is + Why You Want It

> *"Changing long-held negative behaviors, beliefs, and attitudes is challenging. Making big changes can also be a lonely road—but not if you have a health coach to hold your hand, guide you on the path and keep you accountable. With a healthy-living advisor to help you trade old habits for new ones, you won't have to go it alone. My advice? Work with a health coach to change your life this year and create your healthiest self ever—it's a precious gift you'll enjoy for years to come."*
>
> — Dr. Frank Lipman, Integrative Medicine Practitioner and IIN visiting teacher

As a health coach, it's part of my job to have a working knowledge of the types of support available and to understand which one might be right for you. This makes hiring a health coach a great first step! There are thousands of health coaches successfully practicing in all 50 states and around the world. Health coaching includes educating clients about healthy eating and lifestyle choices, helping clients develop and set goals, and taking clients' good intentions and putting them into practice. Health coaches work in many settings and, among other services, provide general wellness and nutrition information, options, recommendations, guidance, motivation, and skill building to establish healthier lifestyle routines to achieve your personal health goals.

Thanks to modern technology, it's easier than ever to work wellness into your life, so don't let your jam-packed schedule stand in the way of you reaching out for support. Like me, many coaches offer a variety of ways to work with them including in person, on the phone, over Skype, or through virtual coaching programs. If finances are an issue, many insurance companies now offer coaching programs, sometimes with reduced premiums or gift cards as incentives. Talk to your company's HR director to find out what type of wellness benefits might be available to you.

## Functional Medicine: Health Care vs. Sick Care

> *"I believe that a healthy person has the most important ingredients to their health built into their system. Our health is an expression of the ability to be self-regulating. When it's time to eat and when we've had enough, when it's time to rest and when to act, etc., are all senses that we are born with. Through our traumas, pathologies and stresses, these messages can get overlooked and eventually become disturbed enough so that we stop living according to them. One way of assessing the health of a person is how well this aspect is working. Accordingly, treatment would be directed to re-establish this aspect of a person as a guide to the success or failure of treatment, and not just the cessation of symptoms. My job then is to track the person's health and to re-calibrate one's systems when necessary."*
>
> — Jonathan Gavzer, LAc, Functional Medicine Practitioner

Many doctors who have trained in the allopathic model of medicine view health as simply the absence of definable disease. By shifting the traditional disease-centered focus of medical practice to a more patient-centered approach, functional medicine addresses the whole person, not just an isolated set of symptoms. Functional Medicine Practitioners (FMP) spend time with their patients, listening to their histories and looking at the interactions among genetic, environmental, and lifestyle factors that can influence long-term health and complex chronic disease. In this way, functional medicine supports the unique expression of health and vitality for each individual. If this sounds ideal, it is!

Working with an FMP can help shed light on unanswered health questions that fall through the cracks of our standard care model. While conventional medicine and functional medicine employ the same diagnostic tools, the key difference is in the interpretation of the information and the treatment protocols that ensue. I learned this firsthand during my own health crisis when after running a full blood panel, an EKG, and pulmonary function tests, my Primary Care Physician (PCP) was unable to determine what was causing my debilitating (and sometimes frightening) symptoms. On your labs, there's a reference range that tells you what is considered "normal," and anything outside this range is typically labeled as "high" or "low" in bold font. That reference range is determined by a statistical bell curve average of the population of that particular lab. If your lab is just one number away from being outside of the reference range, you're still classified as "normal." By using a different assessment of the test results and ranges used, my FMP recognized that my red blood cell count was low. Using that information as our starting point, we did further functional lab work which revealed both adrenal fatigue and absorption issues. A change of diet, lifestyle modification, and a targeted supplement protocol quickly put me back on the path to optimal health. You can find a functional medicine doctor in your area on the functionalmedicine.org website.

## Chiropractic: Mind-Body Adjustment

> *"A well functioning nervous system is essential in creating optimal health. As a chiropractor, I understand the human body is better able to deal with stressors when there is balance in the spine, allowing the nervous system to work free of any structural interference. When the vertebral joints lose proper alignment, it affects how the brain communicates with the body, altering the firing pattern in the central nervous system. The focus of chiropractic care is to keep the vertebrae in their proper relationships with each other, enhancing the function of the spine and nervous system, allowing you to express your full potential."*
>
> — Dr. Jacalyn G. Buettner, DC

Chiropractic is a method of health care based on the premise that good health and mobility rely on a functioning nervous system and healthy spine. Chiropractic allows the body to heal itself by reestablishing communication between the brain and every tissue and organ in your body. This improves skeletal, muscular, and nervous system disorders, often without the use of drugs and surgery.

You might be surprised to learn that the support available to you through a doctor of chiropractic goes well beyond physical adjustments to include the tools you need to maintain whole-body health. Many chiropractors offer nutritional support, detoxification programs, stress management, and physical rehabilitation. Look for word-of-mouth referrals or visit the American Chiropractic Association's website at acatoday.org.

## Holistic Dentistry: Whole Body Health

*"As a holistic dentist, my approach to your health extends beyond dental care. I will work with you to optimize your nutrition, diet and mental and physical well-being. I help my patients become educated, empowered, and active participants in their whole body health."*

— Dr. Nammy Patel, DDS

In chapter six I shared my favorite tips for your pearly whites. I also shared that one of the best things you can do for your overall health is to have any amalgam fillings (carefully) removed. Mercury vapor is a huge source of toxicity, and it vaporizes off amalgams 24/7. I considered it a gift from the Universe when I learned that IIN guest teacher Dr. Nammy Patel opened her holistic dentistry practice right in the heart of Union Square in San Francisco, where I was living at the time. I have Dr. Nammy to thank not only for removing my amalgam fillings, but also for educating me about the whole body benefits of a healthy mouth. You can search for a holistic dentist in your area through the International Academy of Biologic Dentistry and Medicine website (iabdm.org). IABDM is a network of dentists, physicians, and allied health professionals committed to integrating body, mind, spirit, and mouth in caring for the whole person.

## Energy Medicine: Pick Your Woo Woo

> *"I believe in the power of the individual to heal. Balance, perspective and resilience are key components of emotional and physical well-being, and are central themes of treatment in my practice to help clients overcome life's curveballs."*
>
> — Jennifer Brinn, certified Reiki Master and Teacher

In chapter four I introduced you to a whole wide world of woo woo. While there are endless ways to explore energy medicine on your own (and I hope you do), it can be deeply beneficial to work with a qualified practitioner. There are numerous modalities to choose from, but my personal go-to's are acupuncture, Reiki, and EFT Tapping. If you are already working with a health coach or FMP, they will certainly be able to support you in finding someone to work with. In fact, they may even be that person. I found EFT Tapping and Reiki to be so personally beneficial that I incorporated them into my coaching programs, and it's not uncommon for an FMP to also be an acupuncturist.

You know I'm a huge fan of Tapping, but when I first started using the technique I felt a little awkward making up my own Tapping scripts, and sometimes this prevented me from Tapping at all. Luckily, I found Nick Ortner's website (thetappingsolution.com) to be a fantastic resource for easy-to-follow scripts, which I still rely on from time to time. There is also a handy "find a practitioner" link on the site that you can use to find EFT practitioners around the world that you can work with one-on-one via phone, Skype, or in person.

## Therapy: Keep an Open Mind

> *"We're already built, internally on a psychological level, to push difficult thoughts and feelings away. Mechanisms like depression and denial are part of our standard operating system—but healing our lives (and becoming the people we want to become*

*in the process) requires grappling with these internal forces so that we can truly see ourselves and our lives with clarity."*
— Dr. Leslie Carr, Clinical Psychologist

We tend to tell the people around us any number of physical ailments we struggle with, yet we aren't having these same conversations when it comes to our mental health. A tireless advocate for the mental health community, Mama Ruth spent her career supporting people living with mental illness—an isolating disease that affects not only the person with the diagnosis, but the people who love them as well. She made certain that the shame and stigma that can exist around mental illness didn't exist in our home by keeping mental wellness part of the conversation. Stigma harms the 1 in 5 Americans affected by mental health conditions by shaming them into silence and preventing them from seeking help. I'm certain our open conversations made finding support for my disordered eating feel like a natural first step. It also allowed me to see my father's struggles with addiction as a symptom of mental illness—a compassionate view that was instrumental in my own healing.

You don't need a diagnosable mental illness to benefit from seeing a mental health practitioner. If you aren't going to therapy when you think you need it because you feel like traditional talk therapy isn't your thing, you might be happy to know that there are a lot of different options out there and one of them could be perfectly suited to you. I personally love old-school time on the therapist's couch, but it's not the only way to go. There is no one-size-fits-all approach to therapy, and while word-of-mouth referrals can be a great place to start, keep in mind that the professional that works well for someone else might not work as well for you. When researching possible therapists, their website should communicate what kind of approach they take to therapy, as well as information about their education, certifications, and specializations. You can verify a therapist's credentials on the Department of Consumer Affairs website for your state.

If you're on the fence about one-on-one therapy (or even if you are in therapy), you might consider joining a support group or attending workshops that address your most pressing issues. I work with my own therapist in person, by phone, and more recently through Doxy.me, an HIPAA-compliant videoconferencing tool. While weekly therapy isn't a quick fix, finding a supportive person to help you navigate the tricky parts of life is a gift worth giving yourself. You also get to decide if a therapist isn't for you, so don't let one (or more) bad experience in your past hold you back from getting the support you need. I had an unfortunate experience with a therapist in my early twenties, and it was years before I felt ready to try again, but I'm grateful that I did. Know that you are free to consciously uncouple from your therapist.

## Feed Your Mind. Mind Your Feed.

> *"Your ability to be the person you want to be and to live the life you want to live may require that you learn how to be alone with yourself; to leave your house without your phone; to go on a walk with nothing but your own thoughts to keep you company."*
>
> — Dr. Leslie Carr, Clinical Psychologist and mindfulness expert

I am both a student and teacher of mindfulness-based practices, but that doesn't mean that mindfulness always comes naturally to me (that's why it's called a practice). When my friend Dr. Leslie Carr told me she had just finished taping her MindBodyGreen.com course "How to Live Mindfully in the Digital Age," I was excited to support her and (of course) super interested in the topic of mindfulness. Curious about my own relationship with technology, I was not at all surprised to learn that our digital world impacts our thought processes in ways that can sabotage our intentions to create lasting change in our lives. Specifically, it inhibits our ability for self-refection, hinders our ability to be present with ourselves, and impacts our ability to make and carry out long-term plans because as Leslie explains, we are increasingly distracted, overwhelmed, and anesthetized.

While I had a sneaking suspicion that my own behavior with technology had an addictive component to it, it wasn't clear to me why. As it turns out, whether it's a text from a friend or a new like on your Instagram photo, these alerts stimulate the release of dopamine in the brain—the same rewarding neurochemical that's released when a person uses cocaine. I'm still amazed at how easy it can be to trade one addiction for another! Technology can be a particularly tricky relationship to navigate, because our modern lives have made it a necessity. The pull to distract and numb yourself can be strong, and technology provides seemingly endless ways for us to do just that.

Leslie's class not only taught me how to have a healthy relationship with my smartphone (no small task), but it introduced me to an avenue of wellness that's literally at your fingertips. Mindbodygreen courses (www.mindbodygreen.com/courses) offer you an opportunity to learn just about anything wellness from world-class experts, plus it's a great way to explore a topic of interest without making a huge financial commitment. Using technology in this way is one mindful step you can take toward finding more balance in your body, mind, and spirit.

## Closing Meditation: Planting Seeds of Change

In your mind's eye, begin to visualize what the perfect soil for new growth would look like to you. Imagine what this soil would feel like if you held it in your hands. What is its texture, its color, its smell? Imagine that you are tilling this soil, preparing to plant a seed that will grow deep roots. Take a long deep breath and imagine you are lovingly placing this seed into the fertile soil. Cover the seed and water with care.

Focusing on your intention, begin visualizing the change that you would like to see within yourself. Visualize the delicate beginnings of new growth blossoming out of the soil. Imagine this new growth—sturdy, strong, and vibrant. Take another long deep breath as an image begins to take form. This new growth emerging from the fertile soil that you so lovingly tended is you! Once you are able to give form to this vision, take another long deep breath and as you exhale, imagine this new form in its entirety. Observe the details in a way that really allows you to connect with the feeling of what this change would mean for you. You've planted the seeds of change, and each breath you take brings you closer to expressing your full potential ... I'm rooting for you!

# Inspiration & Recommended Reading

I called upon many dear friends, my personal wellness team, and admired wellness practitioners for their words of encouragement and insight while writing this book. It has been my privilege to share teachings that I have received from these dedicated and inspired experts.

Jonathan Gavzer, Functional Medicine Practitioner

Leslie Carr, Clinical Psychologist

Ana Noles, Clinical Psychologist

Jennifer Brinn, Reiki Master

Dan Abels, Acupuncturist

Jacalyn Buettner, Doctor of Chiropractic

Nammy Patel, Holistic Dentist

Shelley Constantini, Certified Aesthetician

Darcy Hunt, Certified Aesthetician

Rosalyn Fay, Women's Mentor & Creator of the Redwood Rose line of products

Alexandra Jamieson, Author, Coach, and Founder of Her Rules Radio

Erin Stutland, Author, Coach, and Fitness Expert

I'm an avid reader and found both inspiration for this book, and wisdom, from the following pages:

Nina Planck, *Real Food*

Debbie Ford, *The Best Year of Your Life*

Christiane Northrup, MD, *Goddesses Never Age* (and every single other book she has written)

Donna Eden, *Energy Medicine for Women*

Alejandro Junger, *Clean & Clean Gut*

Alexandra Jamieson, *Women, Food & Desire*

Nick Ortner, *The Tapping Solution*

Jessica Ortner, *The Tapping Solution for Weight Loss & Body Confidence*

David Wolfe, *Superfood*

Jena la Flamme, *Pleasurable Weight Loss*

Shakaya Leone, *Naked Beauty*

Saida Desilets, *Emergence of the Sensual Woman and the Illustrious Jade Egg*

LiYana Silver, *Feminine Genius*

Naomi Wolf, *Vagina*

Regena Thomashauer, *Pussy: A Reclamation*

Amy B. Scher, *How to Heal Yourself When No One Else Can*

Danielle LaPorte, *The Desire Map*

Joshua Rosenthal, *The Power of Primary Food*

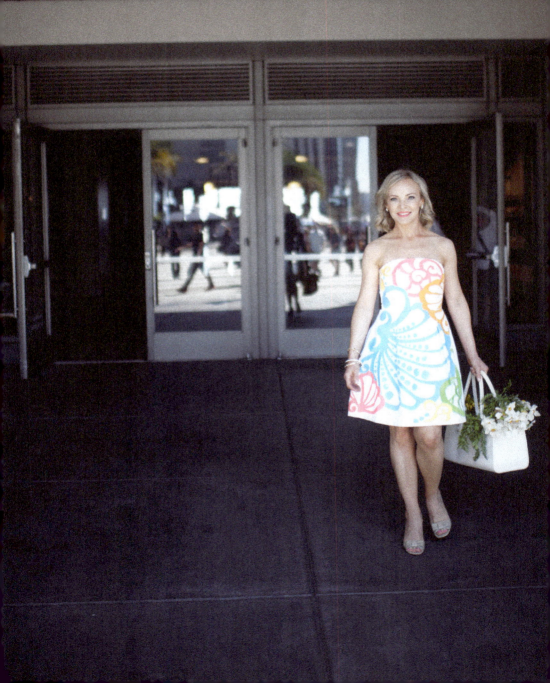

# About the Author

Heather Hudak is an Integrative Nutrition Health Coach certified by the American Association of Drugless Practitioners, Reiki healer, and Ho'oponopono mentor in private practice in Rancho Santa Fe, California. A passionate Wellness Warrior, her mission is to inspire the women she serves to step out of their stories, examine old patterns and beliefs that keep them stuck, and finally step into the lives they were meant to be living. In keeping with her dedication to holistic healing, Heather's programs incorporate a unique blend of nutrition and lifestyle coaching, energy healing, and the co-creation of sacred space in the client's home, providing a nurturing and rejuvenating environment to support women in reclaiming their vibrant health and radiant beauty. You can find Heather on Facebook, Instagram (@happyhudak), and on her website, heatherhudak.com.

CPSIA information can be obtained
at www.ICGtesting.com
Printed in the USA
LVHW070308040220
645781LV00019B/305